A Woman's Guide to
Male Menopause

A Woman's Guide to Male Menopause

Real Solutions for Helping Him Maintain Vitality and Virility

Marc Rose, M.D.,
M. L. Block,
and Virginia Hopkins, M.A.

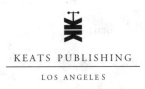

KEATS PUBLISHING

LOS ANGELES

NTC/Contemporary Publishing Group

The purpose of this book is to educate. It is sold with the understanding that the publisher and author shall have neither liability nor responsibility for any injury caused or alleged to be caused directly or indirectly by the information contained in this book. While every effort has been made to ensure its accuracy, the book's contents should not be construed as medical advice. Each person's health needs are unique. To obtain recommendations appropriate to your particular situation, please consult a qualified health-care provider.

LIBRARY OF CONGRESS CATALOGING-IN-PUBLICATION DATA
Rose, Marc R.
A woman's guide to male menopause: real solutions for helping him maintain vitality and virility / Marc Rose, M.L. Lowenstein, and Virginia Hopkins.
        p. cm.
Includes bibliographical references and index.
ISBN: 0-658-00386-0 (pbk.)
        1. Climacteric, Male—Popular works. 2. Middle aged men—Health and hygiene. I. Lowenstein, M.L. II. Hopkins, Virginia. III. Title.

RC884.R65 2000   00-021042
616.6'93—dc21   CIP

Published by Keats Publishing
A division of NTC/Contemporary Publishing Group, Inc.
4255 West Touhy Avenue, Lincolnwood, Illinois 60646-1975 U.S.A.

Printed in the United States of America

International Standard Book Number: 0-658-00386-0

00 01 02 03 04 VP 18 17 16 15 14 13 12 11 10 9 8 7 6 5 4 3 2 1

CONTENTS

ACKNOWLEDGMENTS

Many thanks go to Virginia Hopkins for overseeing all parts of the creation of this book and for her commitment to excellence. Thanks also to our twins, Michael Rose, M.D., and Evan Lowenstein, for their lifelong support and friendship. Much appreciation goes to our editor, Peter Hoffman, for recognizing the unique value of this book and for patiently nudging it along through the editing process.

INTRODUCTION

This book was written for women about men's health, because even in the new millennium, it's almost always the woman in the family who seeks information on health and then applies it. And, fortunately, the man tends to listen when the woman of the family makes a health-care decision. As an anti-aging specialist who has successfully worked with many men over fifty to improve their health, I want to emphasize that the most important steps are the simplest ones: good diet, clean water, exercise, and stress management. The supplements and hormones can make a big difference, but there's no substitute for the basic foundation of a healthy lifestyle. At the same time, a less-than-perfect lifestyle should never be an excuse not to begin changing things today. *Now* is always the best time to begin improving our health, and anything a man does to improve his health—no matter how small a step it may be—is a good beginning.

I couldn't have completed this book without the able assistance and co-authorship of medical writer and researcher Melissa Block, who put my ideas together in a clear, organized fashion and tirelessly tracked down statistics and research. Her educational and professional background in exercise physiology and nutrition was invaluable as we worked to make this information as user-friendly as possible.

You don't necessarily need to sit down and read this book from cover to cover, although we do suggest that you begin with my Eight Steps to Staying Power for Life, and go from there to specific health problems. However, the more you do read, the better you'll understand the aging process and the very specific ways you can simply, safely, and naturally address almost any health concern.

The studies cited in the book are listed in the back of the book, under each chapter, in alphabetical order.

1

Is Male Menopause a Myth?

By the time I was in my mid-forties, I had accomplished a great deal and had had a reasonably good time doing it. I had a thriving ophthalmology practice with my twin brother, Michael. I was fit and healthy and kept up with the latest developments in research on nutrition, exercise, and supplements. I had always taken pride in my trim build. Sometimes I worked a little too hard and didn't take enough time off, but only because I loved my job.

As my fiftieth birthday got closer I started to notice some subtle changes in myself. I gained weight around my middle and more tufts of hair were appearing in my shower drain every morning. My sex life became less and less satisfying, especially for my girlfriend; and after a few unpleasant battles, I didn't even feel like trying anymore. Worst of all, I felt that I was getting old, that my virility and energy were slipping away.

One bright fall morning, not long after I turned fifty, I woke up at six in the morning just as I had for years. My usual routine was to bounce up from my bed and dive into the whirlwind of the day, excited about my work and about life in general. That morning felt distinctly different, though. I didn't want to get up and go to work. I couldn't really think of anything I wanted to do. I felt exhausted, depressed, and old. From that day forward, things kept on going downhill. My irritability, mood swings, and forgetfulness escalated and gave me (and those who had to deal with me) considerable anxiety. Work no longer held any fascination for me, and I trudged through each day without my old sense of purpose. My relationships with loved ones became strained. The life I had worked hard to build seemed empty.

I went to my physician and had a complete physical, hoping to find some answers. I told him about some articles I had read about male menopause, and wondered if that might explain what was happening to me. He chuckled and handed me my "completely normal" test results. "There isn't any such thing as male menopause," he said. "You're just going to have to accept that you're getting older. You can't expect to stay young forever." I walked out of his office with resolve, knowing there must be more to it.

Five years later, I can say with complete confidence that he was wrong and I was right. Male menopause exists. After much research and experimentation, I've put together a program that really works for me and that I now know works for other men as well. I look and feel years younger than other men my age. My zest for life has returned, my work thrills me again, and I have the physical and mental strength and endurance I thought I'd lost forever. I'm even my old self in the boudoir again. At this rate, I expect to be going strong into my eighties and nineties, healthy, strong, alert, and virile. My secrets are all in these pages. If the man in your life feels the way I felt, you can help him rejuvenate himself the way I did. If you're willing to help him make a few changes now, the years ahead have the potential to be the most fulfilling you've had together so far.

MALE MENOPAUSE: FACT OR FICTION?

A woman going through menopause may have hot flashes, night sweats, and significant weight gain. She may have years of erratically fluctuating hormone levels, eventually followed by a drop that causes her to stop having monthly menstrual cycles. Some women coast through menopause without much trouble, while others are plagued with symptoms for years.

Men who have watched this whole process, or who are in the middle of helping a loved one through it, may have breathed a sigh of relief that they don't have to go through it themselves. Still, these same men know they've been feeling not quite themselves lately, either. Maybe he suddenly has a paunch he can't get rid of, even with all those sit-ups he does every day. (Okay, three days a week.) When he does exercise, he gets tired so much faster than usual. He's sprouting wrinkles around his eyes and mouth. His hairline is creeping backward as his bald spot creeps forward. The muscles that have always filled out his shirts seem to be shrinking. He's not quite the lion he used to be in the bedroom, and even when he is in the mood there are times the plumbing doesn't work properly. He may be getting up to pee at night, and the quality of your sleep suffers. Maybe he's feeling generally rundown and is subject to aches and pains and bouts of depression. What's going on?

It's a man's very own distinctly male version of female menopause. Although fertility may not be dramatically affected, the hormonal changes that men go through from their thirties on are significant. Male menopause has a much more gradual onset than female menopause, and so, too often, men with the complaints described above assume or are told by their doctors that these changes are an inevitable part of the aging process.

A woman's passage through middle age may be more noticeable because her hormone levels may drop more rapidly. When researchers cause an abrupt drop in male hormones by giving hormone-blocking drugs, the men being studied actually experience some of the same symptoms women experience at menopause—hot flashes and mood swings included.

I'm going to prove two things with this book: first, that male menopause does exist; and second, that men can keep their energy, their good health, their vigor, their muscle, and their sexual potency into their seventh and eighth decades of life.

However, because the term *menopause* describes the woman's monthly cycles stopping, the term *andropause* (the prefix *andro-* means "male") is a more accurate descriptor of the man's gradual transformation during his forties and fifties. Other names for andropause include *viropause* and *male climacteric*.

Is Andropause the Same Thing As the "Midlife Crisis"?

It's easy to spot the guys going through midlife crisis. They're the ones spending big bucks trying to look good and hide the effects of time's onward march. They're buying sports cars, growing ponytails, and leaving their wives to take up with younger women. Are these previously upstanding citizens going through andropause? Not necessarily.

Andropause doesn't make a man want to go wild, but rather makes him want to take up permanent residence in his La-Z-Boy. It's a physiological change in hormone levels that saps his energy and potency. The midlife crisis, on the other hand, tends to be an emotional or psychological shift. In an attempt to escape unpleasant realizations about aging and mortality, some men "act out" and have a last go at turning back the clock. Potency tends to increase as the unhappy man turns to sex to feel younger. The midlife crisis tends to occur earlier than andropause, in a man's thirties and forties rather than in his forties and fifties.

MALE HORMONES THROUGHOUT THE LIFESPAN

People have been talking about hormones since you hit puberty. You remember puberty: That was when the guys started to feel as though their bodies were composed entirely of erectile tissue, and they started getting interested in contributing their genetic material to just about every female who happened by. Adults, noticing a boy's distracted and secretive air, that dusting of fur on his upper lip, and the outbreak of pimples, smiled knowingly and said, "Ahhh . . . just hormones. Although your man may have gotten rid of the pimples and started to shave, hormones have continued to play a vital role in his body's functioning throughout his life.

The hormonal, or endocrine, system is as finely tuned as the world's best symphony orchestra. Each element is integrated into the whole, and each hormone plays its role just as each musician plays his instrument. The endocrine system's job is to continually produce subtle adaptations in a man's body as the environment he lives in changes. When he eats, exercises, or goes through an illness or stress of any kind, his body senses perceive this, and sensory information is translated by the brain into hormonal messengers that are released into the bloodstream. These messengers, in turn, stimulate other hormonal messengers, until finally the target cells are given the message that they need to grow or change to keep the organism alive.

There are also hormones that are secreted automatically at certain times and in certain amounts each day. This is the body's version of keeping house, making sure all bases are covered and that the organism is functioning optimally.

A college-age man can handle a lot of all-night study sessions, exams, and papers without missing a single keg party because his endocrine system is pumping out hormones that tell the body when and how to repair any damage done by all these stresses. With passing years, however, the glands that make youth-preserving hormones age and start to shrink. The ability of the endocrine system to keep up with all the necessary adaptations slowly dwindles. Suddenly he's in his fifties, not feeling up to par, and looking for answers.

FASCINATING FACTS ABOUT HORMONES

A hormone is a string of protein components (amino acids) linked together in long chains called polypeptides, and is produced and released into the bloodstream by specialized endocrine cells. Glands are basically a bunch of endocrine cells packed together that have the job of manufacturing and releasing hormones in response to the body's needs and in regular daily rhythms. Some hormones cause things to happen in many different kinds of cells throughout the body (growth hormone and melatonin are good examples), while others have very specific actions (such as reproductive hormones like estrogen and testosterone).

Our bodies have figured out a way to make minuscule amounts of hormones and still have them be extremely potent players in the workings of our physiology. Every cell has special receptors for whatever hormones are designed to act on them. These receptors grab onto hormones as they drift by in the blood or body fluids, and pull them in to do their jobs within the cells.

Androgens, for which andropause is named, are one of many types of hormones released by the testicles, and in much smaller amounts from the adrenal glands (small, pyramid-shaped organs that sit on top of the kidneys). About 95 percent of male androgen secretion is from the testicles.

In the womb, all fetuses start out female. When the Y chromosome sends out instructions inside the fetus's body to make androgens, the development of male physiology begins to happen. These high concentrations of androgens cause the fetus to develop the organs that make males male, and also kick in powerfully during adolescence to make males sexually mature.

Androgens also have anabolic effects, which means they cause the growth of muscle, bone, and organs. (The physiques of athletes who use synthetic anabolic steroids vividly illustrate this characteristic of androgens.) Although androgens are considered the "male" hormones, women have them in much smaller amounts in their bodies as well. Men also make "female" hormones like estrogen in small amounts, and you'll see later that some andropausal symptoms are the result of these hormones getting out of balance with the androgens.

Testosterone and dehydroepiandrosterone (better known as DHEA) are the main androgens we'll concern ourselves with in this book. Testosterone is responsible for males' ability to perform sexually, as well as for secondary sex characteristics like body hair, muscularity, and deepening voice. Levels decline steadily from a man's fortieth year on, at the rate of about 1 percent per year. In those at high risk for cardiovascular disease (the number one killer of American males), the decline in testosterone is steeper, which hints at a relationship between this androgen and the body's resistance to heart disease. DHEA is a precursor to many other hormones, including testosterone and the female estrogen hormones. Levels of DHEA peak at about the age of twenty-five and then start to decline slowly, hitting bottom at 10 to 20 percent of peak concentrations in the later years of life. The lower the DHEA levels, the higher the risk of just about any illness related to aging.

I'll go into more detail in later chapters about each of these hormones. The most important thing you need to know right now is that andropause has a lot to do with the gradually declining levels of these and other hormones. Growth hormone, androstenedione, melatonin, pregnenolone, and thyroid hormone also decline with age, and we'll discuss these in detail as well later on. Levels of these hormones are low in old men and in the bodies of those with many of the diseases related to aging. The main thrust of this book is to show how restoring youthful hormone levels is an important step in stopping or even reversing the aging process.

WHY BEING MALE MAKES HIM OLD FASTER

Women live longer than men. This is a well-known fact that is too often accepted at face value, as though women simply have more years in them to be lived. There's more to it than that. Men are much less likely to seek help when they don't feel well than are women. Modern medical treatments for diseases like prostate cancer and heart disease work better when problems are detected early, but men often wait until they absolutely have to seek medical attention. By that time the disease may have advanced too far to be treated effectively. Modern medicine is quite good at patching, drugging, masking symptoms, and doing heroic surgeries that offer quick fixes. For many men, that approach fits beautifully into their way of life, because it lets them get through even severe health problems and simultaneously maintain their stressful, unhealthy lifestyles. But if the root causes of a disease aren't addressed, solutions tend to be temporary. The patient may need another surgery or stronger drugs, he will spend more time feeling lousy, and his lifespan may be shortened.

Men tend to be stoic and deny that they are under the weather at all, and often respond to fatigue by pushing through it. Fatigue is the body's message that something needs more attention and care to function at its best. If that message isn't heeded, the body is subjected to a lot of unnecessary stress. This is physiologically and emotionally damaging and accelerates aging. The less healthy an endocrine system is, the less able one is to cope with that stress, and the problem is compounded. Not only does aging stress us, stress ages us: Research has shown that stress actually can decrease the secretion of the androgens that keep men young and virile.

Although many women complain about having to bleed and suffer cramps and mood swings every month, there is a positive side to this monthly hormonal cycle because they are forced to pay attention to their bodies and deal with their emotions on a regular basis. Men don't have such obvious hormonal cycles, and can go for years and years without ever dealing with difficult emotional issues. The strain of keeping it all inside ages men quickly. Women's menstrual cycles ground them in their bodies, and they can pick up on subtle changes as they happen. That awareness is important in the prevention of life-threatening illnesses.

We've all seen women who seem to lose their minds when dealing with a bout of PMS, and most men have felt lucky that they don't have to deal with that themselves. Look at it this way, though: she gets to release some of the negative energy inside her. The best most men can do is to expend energy in an appropriately macho fashion—perhaps with a game of basketball or racquetball, or manly household chores like shoveling snow or chopping up firewood. Although that may soothe them, the problems that caused the stress to begin with have yet to be healed and will still haunt them. The moral of the story: If you want your man to live a long and healthy life, help him learn to recognize and acknowledge his feelings and, if necessary, help him do the inner work to keep them in balance. This may simply mean being willing to talk things out with you, or it may mean his getting counseling or joining a men's group. Everyone's different. I'll give you more specific suggestions and resources for helping him work with his feelings later in the book.

Staying strong and virile for the rest of his life is not about popping a magical pill every morning and going about business as usual. It's a complete lifestyle overhaul, incorporating mind, body, and spirit with the judicious use of natural hormone replacement. If he (and you) are up for this challenge, you might want to encourage him to start thinking about what he's going to do with those twenty or so additional years he's going to live.

2

Eight Steps to Staying Power for Life

We live in a world that moves at the speed of a sound bite. Possibilities seem limitless. We have access to infinite amounts of information. Advances in technology allow us to send voices and images across continents and oceans at the touch of a button. We have cures for diseases that in previous centuries wiped out entire civilizations. We enjoy comfort and plenty. We can have kung pao chicken delivered to our doors in thirty minutes or less. It's a wonderful time to be alive.

There's a downside to all this lightning-fast progress, however. The human organism doesn't work like technology. It took millions of years of evolution to get us where we are today as a species. The progress of technology is to evolution as a rockslide is to the erosion of stone into sand. Trying to treat our bodies as though they are designed for our fast-paced, fast-food lifestyle can only result in discord. Heart disease, cancer, arthritis, depression, chronic fatigue, and premature aging are some of the ways our bodies revolt against this sort of treatment. All too often we look for the quick-fix solution to our problems. When one part breaks, we patch up that part and hope it holds.

Unlike a piece of machinery, the body consists of dozens of living, breathing, interdependent systems that work together in a precise rhythm that is constantly adjusting itself. If we don't address the underlying systems breakdown that makes us unwell, the delicate balance our bodies so skillfully maintain is tipped. This is how the downward spiral begins into the diseases of aging seen in Western countries.

It's hard to change our ways of thinking and behaving. We are conditioned by advertising to want that which is "fast" and "time saving." Precooked, prepulverized, packaged, and preserved foods line our supermarket shelves. Fast-food establishments offer tasty, filling products, alternatives to taking the time to prepare food at home. Our cars hurtle us at sixty-five miles an hour from appointment to appointment; elevators and escalators carry us up and down; and then we rush to the gym after work to use the latest ab-flattening gizmo.

The Eight Steps to Staying Power for Life are practical guidelines so the man in your life can begin a routine of taking good care of himself, day to day. Without this basic care, nothing else you read in these pages will work to its full potential. The steps are deceptively simple; the real challenge is in making the shift to a more aware, reasonably paced lifestyle. All the basic information given in these eight steps will be addressed in greater detail later in the book.

EIGHT STEPS TO STAYING POWER FOR LIFE

1. MANAGE AND REDUCE STRESS BY CULTIVATING AWARENESS.

Webster's dictionary defines stress as "strain; specifically, force that strains or deforms . . . mental or physical tension, [or] urgency, pressure, etc. causing this."

Some level of stress is inevitable and we need stress in order to thrive. Muscles that are not stressed by exercise deteriorate and droop. A mind that is unchallenged tends to lose its sharpness. But, in excess, stress kills. This is more than an old wives' tale—there's plenty of scientific evidence to back it up.

Heart disease is the leading cause of serious illness and death for American men. Chronic stress during the course of their lives predisposes men to the artery damage that leads to the need for angioplasty at sixty, bypass surgery at sixty-five, and (if the first round doesn't kill them) perhaps another bypass surgery at seventy, with plenty of vitality-robbing medications thrown in along the way.

How do you help the man in your life avoid this fate, starting today? Simply put, he needs to do three things: cultivate self-awareness, have some sort of spiritual practice, and do everything in moderation.

No problem, right? Actually, it's a lot harder than it sounds.

Cultivating awareness means noticing what we do, why we do it, and how we're feeling about it in the process. This is far more challenging to our energy and intellect than going on autopilot. All too often we go into denial about what is hurting us, because we think the situation can't be changed. Not dealing with unpleasant feelings or bad habits takes its toll by causing stress we may not even be aware of. If a man begins to work on noticing what is bothering him on a daily basis, he can deal with it a little bit at a time. This way, taking time to acknowledge and solve problems doesn't stand in the way of his fulfilling his responsibilities.

For example, suggest that the next time he zips down to the vending machine in his office building for a candy bar and a soda, he stop and think for a moment. Suggest that he ask himself if he's really hungry, or if he's satisfying a craving for caffeine and sugar. Is he procrastinating? Is he avoiding being at his desk? Can he think about his body and how good it's been to him over the years? Wouldn't a brisk walk around the block and a bottle of spring water be more in line with what he needs? If he's hungry, he might have some real food—

something with plenty of protein, vitamins, and minerals. If, after serious consideration, he still wants the candy bar and soda, he can go ahead and have it. What's important is that he become aware of what he's doing.

The next step in reducing chronic stress is to engage in some kind of spiritual practice. People who include these practices in their daily routines live longer and recover faster when they become ill. A spiritual practice, such as meditation or prayer, gives you a quiet space and a sense of meaning. Meditation, prayer, yoga, tai chi, chi kung, or a slow walk through beautiful countryside are all spiritual practices that soothe the body and the mind, and provide respite from daily hassles. Encourage him to try a few different practices and see which suits him best. He may soon notice that doing the activity for its own sake expands and intensifies his awareness, nourishing and bringing balance to body and soul.

Keeping a journal can help a great deal. Jotting down ideas, thoughts, and feelings first thing in the morning makes the transition into the busy day easier. Emptying the chatter from his mind onto the paper allows him to be aware without so much clutter in the way. Similarly, writing in his journal before bed can help clarify and resolve issues that arose during the day.

The third component of this first step is about moderation. Americans like radical solutions with immediate gratification. Subtle changes don't work fast enough or noticeably enough to satisfy us. We would rather take powerful prescription drugs than root out the causes of our diseases. We would rather go on crash diets than slowly shift to a lifestyle that doesn't make us fat.

Most quick fixes create imbalance. The body has to swing into a very stressful mode to compensate, and because the body always strives for balance it ends up right back where it started. With weight loss, for example, the faster we lose it, the faster we regain it, and more. More often than not, the body provides insurance against future famine by adding a few extra pounds.

This book isn't about eating nothing but fruits and vegetables, running ultramarathons, or his learning to wrap his legs around his neck. It doesn't endorse bingeing on fatty foods or giving in to the urge to be a couch potato, either. Moderation is the key. Spend Sunday morning on your couch watching TV, but spend Sunday afternoon taking a brisk walk. Have a plate of steamed veggies for lunch, and have your french fries at dinner.

Men's socialization encourages them to think that if some lifestyle modification is good, more must be better. Before either of you clean out your fridge and fill it with trays of wheat grass and bottles of fish oil, before he puts on his (probably somewhat snug) college basketball shorts and goes sprinting out the door for a ten-mile run, realize that this is the rest of his life we're talking about. It can't be an either/or proposition; that simply won't last. Encourage him to ease into these changes and set attainable goals. He needs to listen to his body and take care of it. Macho is out; enhancing performance—mental, physical, and sexual—is in.

2. ENJOY EATING A WIDE VARIETY OF FRESH, NATURAL FOODS, AND CULTIVATE GOOD DIGESTION.

Not only are you what you eat, you're how you eat. If eating is rushed and devoid of sensual pleasure, we may turn to the strong, addictive tastes of fast food and junk food to try to get more enjoyment. Many people say they don't have the time to eat right. It becomes easier to *make* the time once one understands that nothing is more essential for our health and longevity than eating nourishing, natural foods.

We live in an extremely weight-conscious society, and many people make decisions about what to eat based only on the fat content rather than on the nutritive value of the foods. Start to select foods based on their benefits to his and your health. (You'll read about how to do this later in the book.) As he starts to be conscious of the new and wonderful tastes and textures of natural foods while he eats, you'll probably see some of the changes in his body that you've been wanting to see all along.

Whenever possible, choose foods that are the way Mother Nature made them. Fresh, organic produce; organic whole grains; free-range meats; cold-water fish like salmon and mackerel; cage-free eggs; tofu and other legumes; and small amounts of dairy products like yogurt and cheese provide you with a wide variety of choices. It helps when he varies the foods he eats from day to day and season to season. Eating only as much as he needs will also improve his health. He doesn't have to clean his plate. He can learn to avoid sugar, white flour, processed foods, artificial sweeteners, and hydrogenated and unsaturated oils, and to drink alcohol in moderation. For more detailed specifics, refer to chapter 13 on diet.

Both of you need to be wary of fad diets, diet drugs, and supplements about which manufacturers make outrageous promises. If something is advertised as a magical fat-melting, muscle-building, life-extending miracle pill, there's a catch.

3. DRINK PLENTY OF CLEAN WATER THROUGHOUT THE DAY, EVERY DAY.

In his book *Your Body's Many Cries for Water,* F. Batmanghelidj, M.D., makes a convincing case that our species suffers from chronic dehydration. He believes that we could be cured of many degenerative diseases if we would simply drink more water.

Invest in a water filter if you haven't already done so. American tap water is polluted with aluminum; heavy metals; petrochemicals such as benzene, chlorine, and fluoride; as well as with parasites such as *Giardia* and *Cryptosporidium* (which aren't killed by water-plant treatment). Fluoridated water is completely unnecessary for adults and can actually cause harm. Our foods and water contain a lot more of this poisonous element than we need. People with arthritis, heart disease, or osteoporosis should get a special filter to get rid of fluoride in their tap water, and should use a nonfluoride toothpaste. If you would like more information on the hazards of fluoridated water, see the Resources section in the back of the book.

Getting enough water results in clearer, firmer skin, more regular bowel habits, and less appetite for junk food. We also tend to retain less fluid, because dehydration is a signal to the body that it needs to hang onto its water stores.

Only water counts as water, by the way—coffee, tea, sodas, and juices don't go toward fulfilling water requirements. He needs to keep a glass or bottle of water nearby and drink from it often.

4. TAKE NUTRITIONAL SUPPLEMENTS EVERY DAY; AND IF NECESSARY, USE MORE RADICAL TREATMENTS LIKE INTRAVENOUS NUTRIENT SUPPLEMENTATION AND EDTA CHELATION.

More people are using nutritional supplements than ever before. It's becoming more common to use supplements to self-treat mild illnesses like cold and flu (zinc, vitamin C, echinacea, and goldenseal), skin irritations (aloe vera), arthritis symptoms (glucosamine sulfate), and muscle spasms (calcium and magnesium).

Every person, regardless of age, can benefit from the daily use of a high-potency multivitamin. If you, and he, haven't tried nutritional supplements yet, you have a wonderful new world of improving health in front of you. Much of the advice in these pages will include guidelines on what supplements are useful for men going through andropause.

Avoid the store-brand daily multivitamins sold in many drugstores and supermarkets. They contain the U.S. RDA (recommended daily allowance) of vitamins and minerals—the minimum amounts needed to prevent deficiency diseases like scurvy, pellagra, and rickets. I'm advocating optimal health, and that requires taking optimal doses of the vitamins and minerals.

Our modern world is rife with toxins; we suffer from chronic stress; and our food is less nourishing than it was in the days before prepackaging and preprocessing. Our nutrient stores are quickly depleted under these conditions. The science behind the use of large doses of vitamins for the maintenance of health is rapidly advancing, yet there is a great deal more for us to learn. We know that the combinations of nutrients found in foods have yet to be replicated with supplements—in other words, you can't expect to live on junk and take supplements and be in tip-top shape.

For those who are coping with heart disease, diabetes, or other health problems, intravenous nutrient supplementation may be a necessary part of returning to good health. EDTA chelation is another rejuvenating therapy, administered intravenously, that has been used for years by alternative practitioners as a treatment for clogged arteries. You'll learn more about it in chapter 11.

Not many physicians are willing to perform either of these treatments, because they haven't gotten the nod of approval from the American Medical Association, but I'll give you all the information needed to find a doctor who will.

5. Make muscle-building exercise and cardiovascular training a daily habit—but don't overdo it.

We all know that cardiovascular training is important. Brisk walking, jogging, stair climbing, cycling, pickup basketball, swimming, and rock climbing are only a few options. Any activity that gets the large muscle groups of the body working rhythmically for twenty minutes or more, gets the heart pumping, the breath quickened, and the clothes sweaty will do. Every day is best, but three days a week is the absolute minimum.

He also should do some sort of resistance training, with weights, rubber tubing, or his own body weight (as in yoga or martial arts classes), three times a week, to maintain the muscle he has and perhaps build even more. Resistance training is particularly important for andropausal men because it increases levels of androgens and growth hormone. Stretching keeps him limber and protects him from injury.

For those who want to maintain their health and vigor to a ripe old age, none of this is optional! The body was made to move, and when it is forced to sit still day after day, the risk of heart attack, osteoporosis, and some cancers rises significantly.

Many people can't seem to get themselves into a regular program of exercise. They buy gadgets, hire trainers, buy expensive gym memberships, and they find themselves getting burned out and quitting. All anyone needs for a successful exercise program is his own body, a few dumbbells, and some good instruction at the outset.

There are those who push themselves too hard when they exercise, and who overdo it and quit because it never feels good. Very strenuous exercise can hurt by increasing the production of free radicals (see chapter 5), causing injuries, and decreasing resistance against infection. Chapter 6, "Maintaining Muscle for Life," will get him off to a good start.

6. ENJOY AND CULTIVATE AN EMOTIONALLY AND PHYSICALLY HEALTHY SEX LIFE.

Sex is frequently on the minds of most young men, but interest in sex tends to dwindle with passing years. Sex is a wonderful release, a way of being intimate with the important person in one's life, and it feels great. Those who report a healthy sex life live longer and enjoy better health than their counterparts who are less sexually active.

A healthful diet, regular exercise, vitamin supplements, and hormone replacement all add up to greater sexual vitality with passing years. As you'll discover in chapter 7, a man's circulatory, nervous, and endocrine systems all need to be in good working order if his sexual organs are going to work correctly too. Now that so many post-menopausal women are maintaining their libidos with hormone replacement therapies, it's up to the men to keep up with them.

The emotional connectedness that comes along with a good sex life is as important as the physical release of the act itself. Open lines of communication between partners allow both of you to make room for intimacy in your busy lives, and to keep it satisfying for both of you. Strong, trusting relationships with your loved ones are a very important part of the plan described in this book. Does he feel comfortable, safe, and free to express what he's feeling? Or does he feel he's always walking on eggshells, afraid of doing the wrong thing?

Humans are social animals who need others in their lives, working cooperatively to create a community. Studies have consistently shown that people who have pets, who volunteer their time to help others, and who have stable and happy marriages live longer and are sick less often than their less loving and loved counterparts.

Good deeds and heart-to-heart talks can be difficult and time-consuming, but the rewards for making these things a priority are worth it.

7. BEWARE OF DRUGS, UNNECESSARY SURGERY, AND ENVIRONMENTAL TOXINS.

At least 140,000 people die in hospitals each year because of errors in prescribing or side effects of prescription drugs. Billions of health-care dollars are wasted and incalculable damage is done to people's lives. Sounds a lot worse than the street drug problem, doesn't it? I assure you, it is.

I wholeheartedly endorse the judicious use of prescription drugs when they are necessary. Antibiotics, painkillers, and surgeries have saved countless lives and relieved pain for those who would otherwise suffer needlessly. As is often the case with too much of a good thing, however, the indiscriminate and careless use of prescription and over-the-counter drugs carries with it pronounced risk. The problem has gotten so bad that it's getting hard to tell whether a drug is causing or curing an illness.

The good news is that if he follows the advice I'm giving you, he'll need far fewer drugs. Whatever problems he does encounter will likely be treatable with gentle natural remedies. The heroic pharmaceutical and surgical interventions at which modern medicine is so expert will no longer be necessary.

Doctors are just human beings trying to do their job, working against very strict constraints on their time and energy. More patients have to be seen in doctors' offices than ever before just to keep them in business. Physicians' decisions are often based on giving the fastest results in the least amount of time, and this approach encourages the use of multidrug therapy rather than taking the time to discover root causes of the problem. Surgeries to cut out, scrape clean, or otherwise invasively fix what's broken are commonly prescribed, but often are only temporary solutions to problems that require a lifestyle overhaul to remedy.

When you are given a prescription or told that surgery is needed, keep in mind that there are almost always nondrug, nonsurgical alternatives. For an excellent reference on the effects and interactions of prescription drugs, as well as a detailed list of natural alternatives, I highly recommend the book *Prescription Alternatives* by Earl Mindell, R.Ph., Ph.D., and Virginia Hopkins.

Ask the doctor as many questions as you need to feel confident about any treatment prescribed. Seek out your local medical library and read up on options. If you are committed to preventing illness and maintaining health, you may want to shift your primary care to a naturopathic physician or chiropractor.

It's also very important to be aware of the effect of environmental toxins on health. I define *toxin* as any substance that damages the body above and beyond the expected everyday wear and tear of living, and in so doing results in illness or pain.

The human race has made its proverbial bed, and now we're being forced to lie in it. Pervasive, inescapable pollution has spread to the deepest oceans and highest mountain peaks. There's no way to avoid it completely without living in a pod, but you can take reasonable steps by boosting your body's ability to process and dispose of what can't be avoided.

To eliminate major sources of toxins from your life:

- Don't smoke or spend a lot of time around smokers.
- Don't exercise on heavily trafficked city streets.
- Buy organic foods, and stay away from foods that have undergone heavy processing. If you don't recognize or can't pronounce an ingredient on the label, leave it on the shelf.
- Install a good water filter in your kitchen faucet and your shower (chlorine is quickly absorbed through your skin, especially in warm water).
- Don't use pesticides, herbicides, or fungicides. Yes, that means tossing those cans of weed killer and bug spray. There are better, more natural ways to control pest problems.
- Avoid over-the-counter and prescription drugs whenever possible. When you must use them, remember that even something as seemingly benign as a bottle of cough syrup merits a careful analysis of risks, benefits, and interactions with any other drugs you might be using.
- Buy carpets and furniture that have not been treated with chemicals that give off fumes.
- Invest in a carbon monoxide detector, and make sure your home is well ventilated.

8. **As he ages and begins to notice the symptoms of andropause, ask him to have his hormone levels tested and take advantage of natural regeneration therapies including growth hormone, testosterone, and DHEA.**

When I use the term *natural regeneration therapies,* I'm talking about the use of natural hormone replacement and anti-aging supplements that actually turn back the aging clock. Chapters 3 and 4 thoroughly explain which hormones I recommend, and why they work to keep you young. DHEA, testosterone, pregnenolone, melatonin, and human growth hormone are some of the hormones you'll be an expert on by the time you finish this book. Some, like DHEA, pregnenolone, and melatonin, are available without a prescription; others, like testosterone and growth hormone, must be prescribed by a doctor.

Finding a physician who will work with a man on the level I'm recommending in this book won't be easy. Testing for decreasing hormone levels is a tricky business, and some of the standard tests used in physicians' offices won't show deficiencies. (You'll see specifically what tests I mean as you read on.) Many mainstream physicians don't understand why anyone would want to make a distinction between natural and synthetic hormone replacement. It is important to work with a physician who is open to discussion about the patient's needs and who is willing to work *with* him, rather than *on* him.

IN CONCLUSION

These eight steps introduce the chapters to follow and provide a framework, a reference guide you can use as you transform your lifestyle. Any positive changes, however small, will contribute to his better health, greater vitality, and sexual stamina.

3

Men Need Hormone Balance, Too

This chapter will serve as an owner's manual for the male endocrine system. If the man in your life is the kind of guy who reads the manual that comes with his newest electronic or gas-powered gadget from cover to cover, he should find this part of the book particularly interesting. It's pretty amazing that men often know more about how their power tools work than how their own bodies work!

If he is of the "I only read the manual when something goes wrong" ilk, he may be tempted to skip this rather complicated stuff altogether, and may need to shift his thinking a bit to get the most from this book. You can both think of what happens during andropause as similar to what happens to your car when it's time for its 3,000-mile tune-up. Sure, you can take it to a mechanic and leave the whole thing up to him, but we all know how easy it is to get ripped off by a mechanic who knows you don't know how your car works or what it needs. Although there aren't very many physicians who would intentionally give inappropriate or unnecessary treatments, it will help you work with the doctor to keep the man in your life in top condition if you know something about how the male body gets to 100,000 miles with all of its original engine parts.

Once you've read this book you will be well enough versed to understand what is happening to him as he goes through andropause, and he will be able to have educated discussions with his doctor about his plan of care. The better you understand, the easier it will be to help him make the changes he needs to make. Knowledge gives you both the power to make the right decisions.

THE IMPORTANCE OF HORMONE BALANCE

Hormones play innumerable roles in the everyday workings of a man's body. Their complexities are so great that scientists are only beginning to grasp how they work. Lack of a single hormone can make the difference between well-being and life-threatening illness. The body uses hormones to maintain homeostasis (balance) in all its systems despite constant changes in the environment. For example, our bodies go from sleep in a toasty warm bed to rising, bathing, cooking, and eating an assortment of foods. Next we might engage in vigorous exercise, have a conflict with the boss, give a teenage daughter a driving lesson, relax in the sunshine, and see a sad movie. A person working in a stressful profession must work capably while under considerable pressure. All of these activities throw off the body's equilibrium in some way and put a demand on the endocrine (hormone) system to reestablish balance.

There are also rhythms of hormone secretion that aren't based directly on environmental changes, but which are also orchestrated and modulated by the nervous system. Specialized areas of the brain send out signals, daily or several times a day, to stimulate the secretion of some hormones. Hormones are usually secreted at regularly timed intervals throughout the day and night.

STEROIDS: NOT JUST FOR BODYBUILDERS

A man's body is full of steroid hormones. The androgens, such as testosterone, androstenedione, and DHEA; the cortisols; and even pregnenolone, progesterone, and the estrogens, are all *steroid* hormones.

These are different from what you may know as the steroid hormones that bodybuilders take to build muscle. Those are synthetic pseudohormones made in laboratories specifically for their muscle-building qualities. They have very powerful effects, but do not interact gracefully with all the other systems of the body as do natural hormones. In fact, the pseudohormones have unpleasant side effects such as shrinking the size of the testicles and causing acne and "'roid rage."

The natural steroid hormones in men's bodies all share the same basic structure or chassis, with a few pieces that are added or subtracted to change or refine their physiological role. They are all made from cholesterol, which is converted to pregnenolone, which is then converted to the other hormones. (See Figure 3.1.) Some are made in the adrenals; others come mainly from the testicles.

The steroid hormones DHEA, androstenedione, and testosterone are androgens, or male hormones. They are present in women also, but in much lower concentrations. Pregnenolone and progesterone are precursors to many of the other steroids, including aldosterone (an adrenal hormone that governs water balance), cortisol, and DHEA.

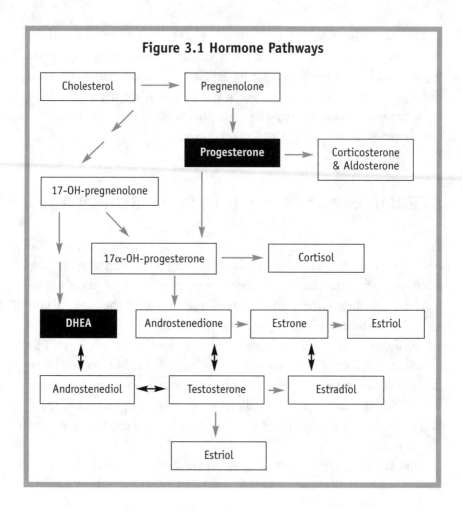

Figure 3.1 Hormone Pathways

The Neuroendocrine System

We can't talk about any of the systems of the body without at least touching on some of the others. Especially well connected are the nervous system and the endocrine system, so much so that they are often referred to together as the *neuroendocrine* system. The *hypothalamus* is a part of the brain stem that is the interface between the brain and the glands. When anything in your universe changes, that information comes in through the senses and is transmitted to the hypothalamus. Daily "maintenance" secretion of steroid hormones is partly controlled by the hypothalamus. Hormonal cycles—regular, day-to-day hormonal needs—and any extra requirements stimulate the hypothalamus to secrete one of many *releasing hormones,* which flow through blood vessels directly to the *pituitary* gland.

Secretion of many hormones also depends on a phenomenon called *feedback inhibition.* Sensors in the hypothalamus perceive that levels are too low and pump out more releasing hormones, and the glands make more of their hormones in response. When levels are within normal limits, releasing hormones stop coming and the gland shuts down or decreases its production. (This happens without the hypothalamus as intermediary in some cases.)

The pituitary gland sits below the hypothalamus, nestled in a pocket of bone within the skull. Often referred to as the "master gland," this two-lobed endocrine organ is attached to the hypothalamus by a thin stalk rich in blood vessels. Each lobe of the pituitary secretes different hormones in response to stimulation from hypothalamic releasing hormones.

For our purposes, we only need to talk about those that come from the *anterior* (front) pituitary. Follicle-stimulating hormone (FSH), luteinizing hormone (LH), thyroid-stimulating hormone (TSH), growth hormone (GH), prolactin (PRL), and adrenocorticotropin (ACTH) all are produced in the anterior lobe of the pituitary gland. When these hormones are released into the bloodstream, they travel to all the tissues of the body and latch onto receptors.

Triggering of these receptor sites causes the cells throughout the body to respond in different ways. Follicle-stimulating hormone causes sperm production in the testicles; luteinizing hormone causes the secretion of testosterone from specialized *Leydig cells,* also in the testicles; thyroid-stimulating hormone causes the thyroid gland to secrete its hormones; growth hormone has effects on all the body's tissues, renewing and repairing the body; and prolactin has the effect of stimulating milk production in the female breast, but is also secreted by men for purposes we don't really understand.

As scientists study the aging process, they are finding that levels of nearly all our hormones drop with passing years. Many of the diseases that affect aging people coincide with the dropping-off of hormone production. Glands age with passing years, and the endocrine tissues of elderly people are usually shrunken and contain deposits of minerals and wastes that inhibit their functioning. In the forties and fifties, right around the time men start to notice symptoms of andropause, this process is just starting to accelerate. The judicious use of hormone replacement therapy to restore youthful levels of hormones in the body can help a man stay healthy and vibrant.

In an ideal universe, we wouldn't need supplemental hormones. The systems developed over millions of years of evolution could continue to do the job just fine. Our universe being less than ideal, small amounts of *natural* hormone supplements can be safely used to help our bodies function optimally. It's important to make this distinction between "natural" and synthetic hormones. *Physiologic* doses of hormones are very small, only enough to restore balance. They are approximations of what the body itself would secrete under ideal conditions, and are much safer and work better than *pharmacologic* doses of many times what the body would make itself.

The typical medical model advocates the "more is better" philosophy, which in the case of hormones is not only ineffective, but counterproductive. Hormones are powerful agents designed for very specific use. The high occurrence of negative side effects in many medical studies of hormone replacement has a lot to do with the use of pharmacologic dosing (often with synthetic versions of the natural hormones our bodies make). Our recommendations involve only physiologic doses of the natural hormones. Moderation brings balance and harmony.

TESTOSTERONE

In 1849, a German physiologist removed the testicles of two roosters and implanted them into the bodies of two other roosters. The castrated roosters became lazy and fat, while the four-testicled ones became, well, cockier—they strutted and chased hens with great vigor, and their combs grew larger and became redder. During World War I, researchers cured a wounded soldier's gangrene by transplanting the testicles of a dying soldier into his body. They also discovered that supplemental testosterone could be used as therapy for intermittent claudication (a painful disease caused by clogged blood vessels in the legs) and for angina (heart pains, also caused by stopped-up blood vessels). In the early 1950s, research showed that testosterone could increase lean mass, including bone and muscle. Aside from making a man look good in a Speedo, this process is important for his body's ability to repair damage as it happens, a little bit every day. Research done from the 1960s through today has confirmed that cholesterol is lowered, abnormal heart rhythm normalizes, symptoms of diabetes improve, and body fat decreases when testosterone levels are supplemented.

Men with low total testosterone are at greater risk of having high levels of fats in the bloodstream (high triglycerides and low-density or "bad" cholesterol, and lowered high-density or "good" cholesterol), being overweight, and having high blood pressure—all predisposing factors for heart disease, the number one killer of American men. A man with low testosterone levels is much more likely to become diabetic. Testosterone replacement can reverse a condition called *insulin resistance,* which is the push that activates diabetic symptoms. Diabetes predisposes a person to heart attacks, strokes, and eye and nerve damage that can lead to blindness or limb amputation. Since testosterone plays a major role in keeping a man's bones strong, low levels of testosterone also put him at greater risk of osteoporosis, the slow weakening and thinning of the bones that affects both men and women.

As men age, they lose muscle and gain fat. Declining testosterone levels are partly to blame for those two or three pounds that mysteriously appear around his middle every year after he turns fifty.

Secretion of growth hormone–releasing hormone (GHRH) from the hypothalamus, and subsequently the secretion of growth hormone by the pituitary gland, is increased by testosterone. Growth hormone is an important youth-preserving hormone discussed in detail on pages 48–56.

Although there is some debate about whether testosterone replacement is a remedy for impotence (see chapter 7 for details), many studies prove that it has the effect of restoring potency, including increasing libido (desire for sex) and frequency and duration of nighttime erections. In a recent study of a group of testosterone-deficient men, testosterone replacement decreased irritability and nervousness and increased alertness, friendliness, energy, and sense of well-being. The memory loss that many assume to be an unavoidable part of the aging process may be reversible with testosterone replacement.

The Message Is Clear: Testosterone Is Good for Your Health

As men age, the Leydig cells of the testes, responsible for making testosterone, begin to die off faster than they are renewed. Total testosterone levels, measurable in men's bloodstreams, decrease at the rate of about 1.5 percent per year. Degeneration of the sperm-making machinery begins around the age of fifty, and the number of sperm samples containing mature sperm decreases significantly. Testosterone levels in young men range from 250 to 1,200 micrograms per deciliter, with ideal levels at least 750 micrograms per deciliter. In elderly men, total testosterone can dip way below the 250 milligrams per deciliter mark.

Although the drop in total testosterone is so gradual that it may not explain the drastic shifts of andropause, the real kicker is the drop in *free testosterone*. As men age, levels of a protein called *sex hormone–binding globulin* (SHBG) increase in the bloodstream. This protein binds with testosterone and makes it unavailable to tissues. It's the free testosterone—testosterone that isn't hooked up with SHBG—that has all the beneficial effects we're talking about. When doctors only measure total testosterone, they may not catch that his free testosterone is low.

As a man ages, his body's mechanism for freeing enough testosterone to keep him youthful begins to fail. Levels of the hormones that stimulate sperm and testosterone production rise along with SHBG as free testosterone levels fall, which is a good sign that the endocrine system senses a lack and is trying to compensate for it.

Testosterone replacement is only available by prescription. I recommend the use of a natural testosterone patch. Don't let the doctor prescribe a synthetic form like methyltestosterone, because synthetics can have some very unpleasant side effects.

I recommend that my patients use enough crystalline transdermal testosterone to restore total blood levels to 900 to 1,200 micrograms per milliliter of free testosterone, and free testosterone levels to 30 to 40 micrograms per milliliter. This dose will vary from person to person, and it's usually necessary to check levels and adjust the dose a couple of times. I prescribe a patch or a gel to be applied to the skin daily.

Monitoring of total and free testosterone levels will allow the dose to be adjusted if needed. It's important to use just enough testosterone to get the benefits and not so much that it causes problems. Too much testosterone can result in acne, a decrease in the size of the testicles, excessive libido, water retention, "testiness" or irritability, and excessive aggressiveness and anger; any of these symptoms indicates the dosage is probably getting too high. An increase in the viscosity of the blood (which raises risk of clogged blood vessels), lowered HDL ("good") cholesterol, and infertility are other side effects that wouldn't be noticed right away, but which will also likely result from getting too much testosterone.

Men with prostate cancer should not use testosterone replacement therapy, and men with prostate enlargement should start with very low doses to be sure it doesn't aggravate symptoms. All men should have a PSA test before starting testosterone replacement therapy (see chapter 8, "Protecting His Prostate").

The next androgen we're going to talk about is dehydroepiandrosterone, or DHEA. DHEA can be converted to testosterone in the body, so a man can try using that first to see if symptoms improve (you can get DHEA without a prescription). Androstenedione, also discussed in this chapter, is also converted to testosterone, and he can try that too if DHEA doesn't help.

DHEA

Dehydroepiandrosterone, or DHEA, is a steroid hormone manufactured in the adrenal glands. These prune-sized glands sit on top of the kidneys and are responsible for the secretion of more than 150 hormones. The adrenal hormones are our major stress buffers, which give us the ability to adapt to whatever stresses our environment brings.

DHEA is the most abundant steroid hormone in the body. It acts as a precursor from which several other steroid hormones are made (see Figure 3.1, page 28), including estrogens and testosterone. Progesterone and the cortisols are made directly from pregnenolone, which we'll discuss shortly. Ninety-five percent of the body's DHEA circulates in the blood joined to sulfur molecules, serving as a reserve that can easily be converted back into the active form.

DHEA production peaks between the ages of twenty and twenty-five, with men having a higher peak than women. There is about a 2 percent decrease in blood levels for each year of life that follows. A large body of research, particularly on men, shows a clear relationship between this progressive drop in DHEA levels and diseases of aging, such as cardiovascular disease, diabetes, and some cancers. In other words, sick people have less DHEA in their bodies than well people do. Elderly people have less than young people, and elderly people with higher DHEA levels are healthier than those with low levels.

Several studies have shown that when DHEA is given to elderly subjects who started out with low levels, there is a sizable improvement in their sense of well-being. Both men and women with some types of cancer, allergies, Type 2 (adult-onset) diabetes, or autoimmune diseases like rheumatoid arthritis have low blood levels of DHEA. This has led researchers to hypothesize that raising DHEA levels can help to prevent or treat these diseases.

Some clinicians have reported success in treating patients who have lupus (an autoimmune disease that can be life-threatening) with DHEA. This androgen may also help prevent heart disease in men, but its effects on heart disease risk in women are much less promising. Most studies on this topic indicate that too high a dose may actually increase a woman's risk, so women should not use DHEA in the quantities that men do.

DHEA aids in the body's immune defenses against unwelcome invaders. One mechanism for this may involve DHEA's opposing actions to cortisol (see pages 39–40 for more about this "fight or flight" hormone). Cortisol is secreted in response to stress, and this has the effect of suppressing the immune system. This makes sense for a caveman. If your body thinks you are in some kind of immediate danger, it doesn't want to waste energy building up the immune system. This would be like deciding to cook dinner in the kitchen of a house that's burning down. Modern life is like the house at a slow burn, where it's too dangerous to really relax and cook a nourishing meal, but not such an emergency that we have to escape immediately. Inescapable, chronic stress leads to constantly elevated cortisol levels, which lessens our immunity against illness. Not only that, but years upon years of overwork can exhaust the adrenal glands, so that cortisol and DHEA levels drop to unhealthy lows.

DHEA supplementation also appears to enhance the youth-preserving effects of growth hormone, which I'll address in detail in chapter 4. This may be one reason behind the remarkable boost of well-being DHEA produces. In one study, a large dose of DHEA given before sleep to ten healthy young men increased the amount of REM (rapid eye movement) sleep. REM sleep is the most restorative kind of sleep and is reduced as we age; the more REM sleep we get, the more beneficial growth hormone we secrete.

Adult-onset diabetes starts out with cells becoming insulin resistant, raising blood sugar above normal levels. In men, DHEA improves insulin uptake by the cells.

To try DHEA, a man should start out with 10 to 25 milligrams daily. Men can take up to 50 milligrams a day, but if he takes that much, it is important to get blood or salivary levels tested at least every six months to make sure he's not overdoing it. (Women should take only 5 to 10 milligrams every other day, because this androgen can have masculinizing effects like the growth of facial hair, acne, and pattern baldness.) Salivary hormone–level checks every six months are a good idea no matter how much one takes. Everyone who uses DHEA should discuss this with his health-care professional and be sure she knows he is using it.

Anyone who has or has had a hormone-sensitive cancer such as breast, testicular, or prostate cancer should avoid DHEA altogether. DHEA is a precursor to estrogen and testosterone, meaning that the body can manufacture those hormones from DHEA. Reproductive cancers seem to be driven largely by the sex hormones estrogen and testosterone, so you should not boost hormone levels when you have those types of cancer. I also don't recommend DHEA for those younger than forty-five unless the levels are measurably low, because it can suppress your natural hormone production.

Please stay away from supplements derived from Mexican yam *(Dioscorea mexicana)* or wild yam *(Dioscorea villosa)*. These products are billed as DHEA or progesterone precursors, which they are decidedly not. Our bodies don't have the enzymes necessary to break down these substances into the steroid hormones. If you want to take DHEA, take DHEA.

PREGNENOLONE

Another steroid hormone made from cholesterol, pregnenolone is the raw material from which DHEA, testosterone, progesterone, the cortisols, and the estrogens are made. It isn't a sex steroid, which means it has no masculinizing or feminizing effects, and it seems to be safe in relatively high doses.

There was a flurry of research done on pregnenolone in the 1940s, but the only clear benefit researchers found was that it relieved symptoms of rheumatoid arthritis. If you suffer from this disease you can try 10 to 200 milligrams divided into three doses daily and see if it helps. It will probably take three weeks to a month to work.

More recent studies show that pregnenolone improves memory after learning, which makes sense if you consider that it has an excitatory effect on the brain. It blocks receptors for GABA (gamma-aminobutyric acid), a neurotransmitter that plays a role in blocking memory. Studies in both rats and humans suggest that pregnenolone enhances the ability to learn and remember. Other studies suggest that it improves sleep and reduces anxiety, and that it promotes healing after spinal cord injury. Pregnenolone appears to play a role in immunity as well, and studies have shown that it can counter the negative effects of excess cortisol (the hazards of which are described on pages 39–40 of this chapter).

Even though pregnenolone is a precursor to all the other steroid hormones, taking a pregnenolone supplement will not necessarily raise the levels of other hormones in the body. It might, but so far the evidence isn't conclusive.

We don't know much about pregnenolone, but I recommend it for my patients who complain that they aren't retaining information when they learn something new, and it does seem to help. You can take up to 100 milligrams daily between meals to improve memory.

ANDROSTENEDIONE

Androstenedione is the direct precursor to testosterone, and appears to have its own important roles in the body. Manufactured in the adrenals and gonads and converted to testosterone in the liver, androstenedione is found in the tissues of many animals and plants. When taken orally, this hormone will raise blood levels of both itself and testosterone, and some report that blood testosterone levels have doubled with use of androstenedione.

Enhanced energy, sexual arousal and function, and sense of well-being have been reported by men who take supplemental androstenedione. In recent years it's become a popular supplement among bodybuilders wanting to increase muscle mass with training by naturally raising testosterone levels. Those who use it report faster recovery times from hard workouts and enhanced muscle growth. What isn't certain is whether the body's natural production of androstenedione or its conversion to other steroid hormones is affected by supplementation.

The conversion of androstenedione to estradiol (one of the estrogens) in bone appears to have a role in keeping bones strong. It isn't known whether it is androstenedione's conversion to testosterone or the precursor itself that is responsible for the bone-preserving effects.

At doses of 50 to 100 milligrams two to five times weekly, adverse effects are unlikely, and you might find it relieves some of your andropausal symptoms.

CORTISOL

Cortisol is the hormone that the adrenals send out when stresses mount. This hormone, while harmful in high concentrations, is absolutely necessary for survival. It's responsible for getting extra fuel in the form of sugars and proteins to the parts of the body that need it. Any stress—including cold, fasting, starvation, infection, intense exercise or emotion, or pain—elicits secretion of a releasing hormone from the hypothalamus that, in turn, brings on cortisol secretion from the adrenals. With chronic stress, the complex feedback system that controls cortisol levels is overridden, and chronically high secretion can cause the gland to grow larger. Adrenal cells begin to die off more rapidly because of this inflammation. Memory, mood, and behavior are all adversely affected.

With advancing years, the feedback system continues to deteriorate, and cortisol levels tend to rise. Too-high levels of cortisol actually cause damage to the parts of the brain that control the body's ability to shut off cortisol release when stress subsides. Chances are good that if cortisol levels are high, DHEA levels are low. This adversely affects immune function, making a person a good target for any bacteria or viruses that happen along. Haven't you noticed that we tend to get sick when we're stressed? Chronically high cortisol levels make it hard to get a good night's rest, and this could be why older or more stressed-out people get less rejuvenating sleep.

Eventually, with years of overwork, the adrenal gland becomes exhausted, and cortisol secretion drops below normal. Cortisol-depleted people feel exhausted and can't cope with the smallest variations from their everyday routines.

If your man is always feeling loaded down with stress, it's important that he learn to deal with it and minimize it rather than trying to keep up a breakneck pace with the help of coffee, cigarettes, or other stimulants. He can take up a meditative practice such as yoga, tai chi, or chi kung. He can get exercise often, but without overdoing it, and enlist the help of a professional to learn productive ways to deal with stress.

Anyone who has been feeling completely wiped out and unable to get through the day may have already exhausted the adrenals, and might need to take small doses of natural hydrocortisone, up to 20 milligrams per day in divided doses. The doctor can administer a salivary cortisol and DHEA test to see if there is a deficiency. Over time, if he follows our dietary recommendations (refer to pages 213–222) and effectively copes with stress, his adrenals can restore themselves and make enough cortisol again.

PROGESTERONE, THE NEUTRALIZING HORMONE

Although we think of progesterone as a female hormone, it's not a sex hormone, so it doesn't create male or female attributes if you take it. This is an important distinction, especially since one of its major roles (aside from being a precursor to all the other steroid hormones except pregnenolone) is maintaining pregnancy. In men, progesterone is made by the adrenals, and it may also be made in the nerve cells. It has important effects nearly everywhere in the body.

Pregnenolone and progesterone are essential parts of the fatty sheath that surrounds nerves. This myelin sheath protects nerve tissue and speeds up transmission of nerve impulses. Rats with spinal cord injury recovered better when given supplemental progesterone.

Although estrogens stimulate cell growth, it is progesterone that signals cells to mature and differentiate. John R. Lee, M.D., an expert on hormones, has revealed an epidemic of "estrogen dominance" in both pre- and postmenopausal women and in older men, where estrogen's effects run rampant because it is not sufficiently opposed by progesterone, and in the case of men, both progesterone and testosterone.

Transdermal natural progesterone cream is being used by some alternative health professionals to treat baldness and prostate enlargement (BPH) in men. I have heard a trickle of reports that it works to grow hair, and many reports that it significantly helps reduce prostate enlargement and its accompanying symptoms. I have also heard reports that progesterone has reversed prostate cancer. Please be aware that this is very experimental. However, the theory is sound: Estrogen stimulates cell growth, and progesterone balances or opposes this tendency.

In the case of hair, excessive estrogen tends to cause hair loss, while progesterone blocks that estrogenic effect.

If a man wants to try using progesterone to treat BPH, see chapter 8. To use it to grow hair, try rubbing on a dab of the cream before going to bed at night. You can find progesterone creams in the women's health section of most health-food stores. Choose a cream that contains 450 to 550 milligrams of progesterone per ounce, and that contains no other active ingredients, except vitamin E.

ESTROGENS, THE FEMALE HORMONES

Estrogens are the most distinctly "female" hormones. Men make very small amounts in their adrenals and fat cells. Men with prostate cancer are often prescribed estrogens to counteract the supposed cancer-promoting effects of testosterone (see chapter 8 on prostate health for more on this therapy), but because estrogen stimulates cell growth, that seems to me to be going out of the fire and into the frying pan. I don't recommend it.

You may be wondering why we're addressing "female" hormone balance in a book on andropause. It's because our environment and our foods are loaded with potent substances known as xenobiotics, many of which have estrogenic effects. Each of us is exposed to these xenobiotics from the time of our conception, and in spite of the government's supposedly rigorous testing of all chemicals deemed safe for use, these chemicals continue to have frightening effects on animals and humans.

Chemicals derived from petroleum (petrochemicals) are a major source of xenobiotics. They are found in pesticides, plastics, furniture, the fiberboard used to panel buildings, and carpeting, for example.

When we sit down to enjoy a dinner of steak and potatoes, we're getting a dose of xenobiotics stored in the cow's fatty tissues and residue from the pesticides sprayed on potatoes, lettuce, and green beans. The plastic wrap put around the potatoes in the microwave can release xenobiotics into the food. These estrogenic chemicals will be stored in our fat or immediately metabolized in our bodies, and will compete with the masculinizing effects of testosterone. Xenoestrogens may also compete with progesterone, affecting the function of the nervous system and the formation of testosterone, DHEA, and other essential androgens. Animal studies have shown that many populations of fish and reptiles are losing the ability to reproduce because of the feminizing effects of petrochemicals on males, and the interference they create in female reproductive organs. The upswing in male infertility could very well be attributable to the same chemicals. It sounds like a science-fiction movie, but it's real.

What can you do? Start by following our dietary guidelines on pages 213–222. The more organic produce and meats you can eat, the better off you are. Don't cook your food wrapped in plastic; don't make a habit of eating food or drinking water that has been stored for long periods in plastic containers. Limit your use of pesticides and chemical fertilizers in the garden. There are some excellent books that can help you limit your exposure to xenoestrogens and other environmental toxins; see the list in Resources.

WHAT TO EXPECT WHEN YOU GO TO A PHYSICIAN FOR HORMONE REPLACEMENT THERAPY

The first thing you should know is that many physicians believe that aging is inevitable, and that we shouldn't bother trying to resist its debilities and diseases. Finding a doctor who practices anti-aging medicine is the first thing to do. A physician who responds to complaints of any age-related complaints with a hearty "What do you expect? You're getting older!" is not the one to consult.

Most physicians who practice anti-aging medicine practice it on themselves. They tend to live healthier lifestyles, keep up with the latest research, and are shining examples of their own expertise in prescribing appropriate doses of hormones and supplements. Anti-aging physicians are willing to work cooperatively with patients over the long haul for the best possible results. For a referral to an anti-aging physician in your area, contact the American Academy of Anti-Aging Medicine at (773) 528-4333.

A physician who practices anti-aging medicine will be able to develop the right hormone and supplement "cocktail" for your man. He will ask questions about how he's been feeling; it is essential that he describe any symptoms in detail.

A series of tests to measure biological age are also in order. Not only do these tests give the doctor guidelines for prescribing HRT, but they also provide baseline data that will allow him to measure improvement after therapy is in place. The doctor may order some or all of the following tests.

FUNCTIONAL TESTS

- Forced vital capacity—a machine called a spirometer is used to measure the power with which you can exhale all the air in your lungs
- Muscle function tests
- Cardiovascular capacity and cardiac testing—usually with a treadmill test at the cardiologist's office
- Kidney function tests
- Neurological/sensory testing—hearing, vision, memory, and reaction time

- Immune function testing—to count the number of circulating immune cells and measure their activity

Biological Tests

- Bone density
- Measurement of skin elasticity—the doctor simply pinches up the skin on the back of the hand and measures the length of time it takes to return to normal
- Measurement of fingernail growth rate—an excellent marker of biological age
- Body composition tests—to measure fat and lean tissue compartments
- Measurement of hormone levels, including DHEA, growth hormone, testosterone, and estrogen; the new salivary hormone tests give very reliable readings
- Measurement of thyroid hormone, insulin sensitivity, antioxidants, cellular coenzyme Q10, and cancer antibodies in the blood

Based on the results of these tests, the physician can make a good guess at what is needed. After starting on replacement hormones, expect to have a couple of follow-up visits for lab values and yearly follow-ups thereafter.

IN SHORT

Hormones do not work alone. They interact and transform, working synergistically to keep us going strong. Not only is it important to keep hormone levels adequate, it's also important to maintain the delicate and complex balance that exists between them. This chapter only touches the tip of the iceberg. The future of hormone replacement therapy (HRT) looks very bright right now, and researchers predict that humans, with the aid of HRT, will be living into their twelfth and thirteenth decades before long. The understanding you've gained in this chapter will help you to take advantage of these innovative therapies as they become more readily available.

4

The Anti-Aging Hormones

Now let's take a look at some other hormones that men's bodies use to regulate the rate at which they age: human growth hormone, insulin, and melatonin.

The synergy of the endocrine system makes it difficult to address each hormone separately. Without the proper balance of hormone levels, no one hormone works to its potential. Here are a few examples of how hormones work to check and balance one another:

- Levels of testosterone and growth hormone are each increased by the other.
- Growth hormone decreases the rate of production of cortisol, the stress hormone produced in the adrenal glands.
- Growth hormone aids the conversion of the inactive form of thyroid hormone (T4) into the active form (T3).

- Melatonin and growth hormone have synergistic effects.
- When insulin and growth hormone levels are both kept in the right range, they check and balance each other beautifully. If the balance is tipped by too much insulin and not enough growth hormone, the consequences are weight gain and possibly adult-onset diabetes—both of which lead to accelerated aging and blood vessel disease. In this chapter, we'll see how to control insulin levels with diet and exercise, and restore youthful levels of growth hormone.

When a comprehensive hormone replacement and enhancement program is in place, your man needs only very small doses to achieve the optimal balance. The interplay of the various elements within his body does the rest.

In this chapter I want to place special emphasis on growth hormone, because, in my opinion, the work being done with it is incredibly exciting and at the forefront of anti-aging research.

HUMAN GROWTH HORMONE

If the man in your life could take a medication that would build muscle, melt away fat, smooth wrinkled skin, strengthen his heart, restore his libido, and make him feel incredibly good, would he take it? You're wondering what the catch is. "Will it kill him in five years?" "Are the side effects severe?" "Does it cost millions of dollars?"

No, it won't kill him in five years, and it looks as though it may prolong life. I'm not talking about extra years in the convalescent home, either—I'm talking about vital, energetic, productive years. With proper dosing, this magical substance has no side effects at all. It is expensive, but doesn't cost millions of dollars—and there are ways to stimulate the body to pump out more of this miraculous stuff if the injections are too expensive.

This miracle elixir I'm referring to is human growth hormone (HGH), a substance secreted by your own pituitary gland. Growth hormone–releasing hormone (GHRH) is sent from the hypothalamus to signal the pituitary gland that there's a need for growth hormone. When the pituitary gland, which sits at the base of your brain, pumps growth hormone into your bloodstream, it stimulates the release of a growth factor, IGF-1 (insulin-like growth factor 1). IGF-1 causes increased protein synthesis in whatever tissues it encounters.

HGH is itself a sort of intermediary—stimulated by GHRH, and in turn stimulating chemicals known as growth factors to go into the cells and carry out their duties. Think of growth hormone as the powerful executive that goes in to work each day, and who gets his orders from above (GHRH). Once it's clear what task he needs to accomplish, he can delegate some of his authority to those working beneath him (the growth factors).

For simplicity's sake, I'll just refer to "growth hormone" from here on, but remember that it often affects the tissues indirectly, delegating its authority. Replacement of GHRH or IGF-1 is being studied to see if their effectiveness as therapy for andropause matches that of growth hormone. Researchers are discovering that GHRH and IGF-1 have a few of their own specialized functions.

GROWTH HORMONE FROM BIRTH TO ADULTHOOD

When a tiny baby makes its astonishing transformation into an adult, it's because the pituitary gland is pumping out huge amounts of growth hormone. If a child has insufficient growth hormone secretion, dwarfism is the result. In recent years, treatment with growth hormone injections has helped these children grow to normal stature. On the other end of the spectrum are pituitary giants—those with pituitary tumors or some other problem that causes out-of-control growth hormone secretion.

The effects of severe growth hormone deficiency in adults, which can result from pituitary tumors or other hormonal disorders, are far-reaching. Life expectancy is reduced, the heart muscle is weakened, metabolic rate slows, muscle and bone deteriorate, fat accumulates, the kidneys don't work properly, skin becomes thinner, cholesterol levels rise, blood sugar regulation is disturbed, amount of restorative sleep decreases, and emotional health is adversely affected.

Think of someone you know who is elderly. Picture him in your mind. Now go back over the list of symptoms of growth hormone deficiency in the paragraph above. Do the symptoms of growth hormone deficiency pretty accurately describe the condition of the elderly person you're holding in your mind's eye?

As we age, our organs shrink and lose some of their function. Our bones become more brittle, our muscles atrophy, and our skin and connective tissues become less pliable. With growth hormone replacement, these changes can be halted and even reversed.

With each passing decade, we secrete about 14 percent less growth hormone. By the time we reach age sixty, we are, functionally, growth hormone deficient. It follows that growth hormone replacement should reverse the deterioration that we've come to expect with aging.

FAT BURNER, MUSCLE AND ORGAN BUILDER

Growth hormone has an *anabolic,* or tissue-building, action in the body. Muscle, bone, connective tissue (tendons and ligaments), and organs replenish themselves in response to HGH stimulation. Fat tissue is the exception to this rule; there is a decrease in the storage of excess calories as fat when growth hormone is secreted, and fat is preferentially burned as fuel.

In one study, investigators found that GH had a shorter duration of action in the bloodstream of overweight subjects, and overall production of GH was only one-fourth that of their normal-weight counterparts. In the same study, obese subjects responded only weakly to powerful stimulants of growth hormone secretion, including insulin;

to the amino acid arginine; and to exercise and sleep. Obese men also tend to have higher levels of cortisol (the stress hormone) and insulin, and lower levels of androgens than thin men. This hormonal milieu sets you up to accumulate even more body fat.

Growth hormone levels especially affect the heart. People who lack HGH because of pituitary disorders are twice as likely to die from cardiovascular disease. Giving GH to patients who are deficient in it increases the pumping strength of the heart. When HGH was replaced in lab rats after they had heart attacks, huge improvements were seen in the openness of blood vessels throughout the body and in the heart muscle's contractility. GH therapy lowers diastolic blood pressure (the pressure of blood pushing out against arteries while the heart is between beats).

Growth hormone is also involved in the upkeep of the kidneys and liver. Replacement therapy brings these organs back to a youthful level of function.

IMMUNITY ENHANCER, CHOLESTEROL CLEANER

Studies are revealing that growth hormone plays an important role in helping the body fight off infection. When GH enters the cells of an important immune system builder, the *thymus* gland, it causes those cells to multiply. Declining growth hormone levels may partially explain our reduced immunity as we age.

Growth hormone also has some interesting effects on the liver. This organ is responsible for producing cholesterol and processing the cholesterol we eat. GH stimulates the liver to grab and "digest" excess cholesterol, which brings blood cholesterol levels down a few notches.

DIABETES AND GROWTH HORMONE

Now that you're discovering how intimately all the hormones are connected, you might guess that diabetes isn't only about insulin. Diabetics have fewer growth hormone receptors, and they don't make as much IGF-1 as people without diabetes. Growth hormone given in pharmacologic (higher than normal) doses to people with normal insulin levels can result in increased insulin release and insulin resistance—in other words, diabetes. Animal studies indicate that if IGF-1 is also given, this doesn't happen. Studies are piling up to support the use of IGF-1 replacement in diabetics to improve insulin sensitivity and reduce blood cholesterol.

C'MON, GET HAPPY

Those who have tried HGH give it the most glowing of reviews. They say it lessens depression, fatigue, anxiety, and irritability, and enhances feelings of well-being and calmness, attention span, and memory. The great improvement in emotional health seen with DHEA replacement may be due in part to the boost it gives to HGH levels.

SIDE EFFECTS EXPLAINED

The key word here, as with the androgens I discussed in chapter 3, is *replacement.* In several studies that administered growth hormone pharmacologically (infrequently, in large amounts) rather than physiologically (frequent delivery of small amounts), there were unpleasant and even dangerous side effects. Bloating from fluid retention, insulin resistance (the beginning of adult-onset diabetes), and carpal tunnel syndrome were seen in subjects of these clinical studies. There is absolutely no reason to expect side effects from growth hormone levels identical to those we had in our younger years.

Secretion of growth hormone from the pituitary is *pulsatile*—that means that there are small bursts in a regular rhythm, and the amplitude of these bursts increases in response to certain stimuli (which I'll discuss below). Dr. Edmund Chein, at his Palm Springs Life Extension Institute, has developed a twice-a-day protocol for growth hormone replacement therapy. His patients inject themselves with small doses right before going to bed and just after waking in the morning. This better approximates the body's natural release of the hormone. When growth hormone is given in this way, there is very little risk of side effects, because you're simply restoring the same levels you had in your youth.

One risk that warrants further exploration is HGH's effect on cancer cells. Tumors, just like other tissues, are stimulated to grow by HGH, and if you have cancer it could be worsened by replacement of this hormone. However, in one promising study of rats given experimental cancers, tumor size markedly *decreased* in animals given GH and a low-protein diet. The stimulation of the immune system by HGH could be adequate to counteract enhanced tumor growth, but more research is needed.

Unfortunately, growth hormone replacement is very expensive right now, adding up to at least thirteen thousand dollars a year. For those who can afford it and who are deficient, I recommend it. If you are interested, speak with your physician.

If it's out of reach, don't despair—there's a lot that can be done to enhance the body's natural production of growth hormone.

HOW TO NATURALLY PUMP UP GROWTH HORMONE SECRETION

Exercise is a powerful stimulator of growth hormone secretion. Certain kinds of exercise are better than others for this purpose. I'll discuss this in detail in chapter 6 on exercise.

The amplitude of growth hormone pulses increases dramatically during deep sleep, as your body uses that time of rest to lay down new, healthy tissues to replace damaged ones. For most people, aging means more difficulty getting a good night's sleep. For pointers on how to improve the quality and quantity of sleep, refer to the section on melatonin in this chapter.

There are also some dietary manipulations to try. Weight loss is a good place to start; as I mentioned earlier, obesity brings GH levels way down.

One of the most powerful stimulators of growth hormone secretion used by researchers is *insulin-stimulated hypoglycemia*—that is, low blood sugar. Fasting causes spikes in growth hormone secretion, and one- to three-day fasts every few weeks are a good youth-preserving tactic. When animals are chronically underfed, they live longer and healthier lives. This probably has much to do with the decrease in oxidative stress that results, but underfeeding also stimulates growth hormone production. Fasting is beneficial for many other reasons—it allows the body to flush itself clean of toxins, and gives the intestines a chance to mend any damage. (Tiny leaks in the walls of the small intestines allow large food particles to escape into the bloodstream, eliciting an immune response and bringing on symptoms of food allergy.) If you're interested in finding out more, refer to Ralph Golan, M.D.'s classic book *Optimal Wellness*.

Studies show that meals rich in protein cause a boost in blood levels of HGH. Certain natural and synthetic amino acids, vitamins, and even some prescription drugs are very potent growth hormone *secretagogues*—in other words, they stimulate HGH release and action.

The amino acid *arginine* is often used in studies to elicit growth hormone surges. Intravenous arginine causes a four- to sixfold jump in blood growth hormone levels! Oral doses don't work as reliably or dramatically. The research shows that if growth hormone is deficient and arginine supplements are taken regularly, growth hormone response is enhanced. That means that during sleep or exercise the extra arginine boosts the body's natural growth hormone response. Lysine, another amino acid, greatly potentiates the effect of arginine on growth hormone levels; optimally they can be taken together. Your partner can try 1,200 to 1,500 milligrams each of L-lysine and L-arginine on an empty stomach, an hour before exercise or an hour before bed. If this is tolerated well, he can try up to 3,000 milligrams of each.

Ornithine, glutamine, and *glycine* are other amino acids that can be combined with arginine to improve its growth hormone–enhancing effects. Ornithine can be converted to arginine, and enters the cells more easily than arginine itself. Clinical studies of glutamine and glycine have shown both of these amino acids to be effective promoters of growth hormone secretion, but more research is needed to establish guidelines for proper dosage of each. Generally, very high doses—from 8 grams up to 30 grams—are used in experiments, and researchers using lower doses have not had consistent success.

Amino acids administered in pharmacologic doses have pharmacologic actions in the body, and that can mean unpleasant gastrointestinal side effects and toxicity. It is important to begin with small doses of 500 to 1,000 milligrams and build up. Vincent Giampapa, M.D., medical director of the Longevity Institute International (LII), suggests "stacking" these growth hormone secretagogues, starting out at 2 grams each of arginine and ornithine and 1 gram each of glutamine and lysine. Build up to 2 grams of all four amino acids.

Gamma-hydroxylbutyrate (GHB) is a substance found throughout the body. When supplemented, it increases levels of gamma-aminobutyric acid (GABA). GABA stimulates the pituitary gland to produce more GH. Anecdotal reports indicate that GHB is a potent aphrodisiac and sleep inducer as well. The side effects of GHB can be serious, including liver damage and seizures, and at this point I can't recommend it as a supplement.

You can also purchase an amino acid supplement called PROhGH (Symbiotropin), an all-natural, plant-based combination of HGH secretagogues. There are quite a few studies to support its effectiveness at boosting GH levels. The tablets contain some synthetic amino acids as well as L-glutamine, L-arginine, L-pyroglutamate, GABA, L-glycine, L-lysine, L-tyrosine, and a natural version of the prescription drug L-dopa (see page 56). It should be taken on an empty stomach at bedtime, or in the morning forty-five minutes before eating. You should be able to find Symbiotropin for sale at your health-food store, at stores where bodybuilding supplements are sold, or on the Internet.

Niacin, the B vitamin, has been shown to boost GH levels when taken in doses of 200 milligrams to 1 gram. Often prescribed as a cholesterol-lowering drug, niacin can cause a predictable hot flash known as the "niacin flush," which may be a little uncomfortable. It is not dangerous, however. To avoid a flush, the dose should start at 50 milligrams and increase gradually.

Several prescription drugs are effective GH releasers. *L-dopa* is usually prescribed to those with Parkinson's disease. *Hydergine* enhances memory and stimulates GH secretion at higher doses. *Phenytoin* (Dilantin) and *clonidine* (Catapres) are other prescription drugs that may soon be prescribed to people over the age of forty to stimulate release of growth hormone.

INSULIN

Gerry is in his fifties, and has struggled his whole life with a weight problem. "I was a fat kid, a fat teenager, and now I'm a fat adult," he sighs when he comes to my anti-aging clinic, weighing in at three hundred pounds. "I've tried every diet there is, and nothing works for me except starving myself. Every time I do that, I feel great and lose a lot, but then I gain it all back. Now my blood pressure is high, and my cholesterol is out of whack."

I ask him what kinds of diets he's tried.

"Oh, you know, mostly the ones where you cut out all the fat."

It turns out that Gerry's idea of being "on a diet" means eating processed "dietetic" foods, breads, pasta, sugary yogurt, diet sodas and juice drinks, and low-fat packaged snacks. There are virtually no nutritious choices on his list of acceptable "diet" foods. I suggest that he try a more balanced approach, eating vegetables, fruit, tofu, and plenty of deepwater fish, and avoiding all foods labeled "diet," "reduced fat," or "sugar-free." As part of his physical, I do a glucose tolerance test and discover that he has subclinical diabetes, a result I fully expected.

THE MANY ROLES OF INSULIN

The pancreas is a gland located along the small intestine. This organ is an endocrine powerhouse responsible for the manufacture and secretion of a few very important hormones, including insulin.

When you eat a meal, your digestive system breaks the food down into its most basic components, which can then be used by your body as fuel. Carbohydrate foods become glucose (sugar), protein foods become amino acids, and fats become fatty acids. Glucose, amino acids, and fatty acids also can be stored for later use. Glucose is stored mainly in the liver and muscle tissues, amino acids are incorporated into the body's proteins, and fats are stored in adipose tissue.

Carbohydrate foods, when broken down into glucose, cause a steep rise in blood glucose levels. This triggers the pancreas to secrete insulin. The main job of insulin is to grab on to the extra sugars and transport them into the cells of the liver, muscle, and fat tissues, where they are used as fuel. The rate at which fat and protein are metabolized is also regulated by insulin, mostly due to its effects on enzyme activity within the cells. Insulin promotes the storage of fat and protein and inhibits fat and protein breakdown. Insulin promotes the use of glucose as fuel and spares fat and protein, directing them to storage.

If insulin is not present or doesn't work properly, blood sugar levels shoot up but the cells can't use any of it. Severe illness and even death soon follow if the problem isn't quickly remedied. This is what happens in diabetes, a disease that wreaks total havoc in the body. If a child has diabetes and needs to use insulin, it's because of some problem with the pancreas. When a middle-aged or older adult becomes diabetic, it's usually due to poor diet, lack of exercise, and being over–weight. Adult-onset, or non–insulin-dependent, diabetes (NIDDM) is at epidemic proportions now, with more than 10 million people affected.

In Gerry's case, for example, his cells had become *insulin resistant.* It seems that in many cases the human body responds to obesity by preventing the insulin from doing its work. Glucose isn't passed into the cells, and blood glucose levels become too high. The pancreas tries to keep up with the rise in blood sugar by pumping out more and more insulin. Hyperglycemia (too much blood sugar) and hyperinsulinemia (too much insulin) set the stage for diabetes.

Under these conditions, the body is forced to rely on stored fats and protein for energy. *Diabetic ketoacidosis* is the result—the byproducts of fat and protein breakdown *(ketone bodies)* collect in the bloodstream, acidifying the blood and slowly poisoning the body. The undiagnosed diabetic finds himself urinating very frequently and suffering from unquenchable thirst and dehydration as excess glucose and ketone bodies are flushed out in large volumes of urine. Adult-onset diabetes can have a very gradual onset, and many cases go untreated until the problem is completely out of hand. Diabetics tend to feel awful all the time, and complications begin to occur very early in the disease process if the problem isn't remedied.

Many people go for years with undetected or borderline (subclinical) diabetes, which has widespread effects on their cardiovascular and nervous systems. The combination of chronic high insulin levels and out-of-control, high blood sugars does terrible damage to the blood vessels throughout the body. High blood pressure, high levels of fats in the bloodstream, heart attack, stroke, eye disease, neuropathy (irreversible pain or numbness in the extremities resulting from poor blood flow to nervous system tissues), and loss of muscle tone in the sphincters of some internal organs can result.

Maintaining good insulin function throughout andropause is a very important part of avoiding heart disease, the number one killer of men. Anyone who is already being treated for hypertension, high triglycerides, or adult-onset diabetes should know that many people eventually wean themselves off the medications prescribed for these disorders when they modify their diets and exercise regularly. I gave you the guidelines in the Eight Steps; also refer to chapter 6 on exercise and chapter 13 on diet.

Recently there has been a surge in popularity of weight-loss diets specifically tailored to keep insulin levels low. Chapter 13 gives the lowdown on the trendiest diets—and how to design a version that works for your man. My nutritional prescription for diabetics includes foods rich in vitamin C and *bioflavonoids,* like blueberries, lemons, cherries, grapefruit, plums, red onions, and raspberries. (Bioflavonoids are necessary for the proper absorption of vitamin C, which is in turn necessary for maintaining the structural integrity of the blood vessels.) Replace all refined sugars and carbohydrates with whole grains and vegetables, and have some lean protein at each meal.

The use of supplements in the treatment of adult-onset diabetes is becoming more and more common. These nutritional supplements have potent balancing effects on blood sugar levels, so if your partner is taking insulin or oral diabetes drugs and wants to try these supplements, be sure to work in partnership with a health-care professional and monitor your partner's blood sugar frequently. Blood sugar changes vary with the individual and by how well the diet and exercise regimen is going. Possible supplements are:

- Chromium picolinate, 100 to 200 micrograms

- Vanadyl sulfate, 10 to 25 milligrams

- Alpha-lipoic acid, 500 micrograms per day in divided doses (it may cause blood sugars to drop, so be prepared)

He can also take 2,000 milligrams of vitamin C, in divided doses, per day. This may alter the color of the urine strips used to measure his blood sugars, so be sure the doctor knows he's taking the supplement. Other helpful supplements include *quercetin,* a bioflavonoid (500 to 1,000 milligrams per day) and magnesium (400 milligrams at bedtime), to manage the high blood pressure common in diabetics. *Omega-3* oils from cold-water fish, garlic, and zinc all work to maintain blood vessel health.

MELATONIN

The tiny pineal gland, located deep within the recesses of the brain, makes minuscule amounts of a hormone called melatonin. (Melatonin is also made in the retinas of the eyes and in the intestines.) The pineal gland uses this hormone every night when it gets dark to put the body to sleep. In rats, daytime melatonin secretion appears to be one way their bodies counteract the negative effects of stress.

As with all the other hormones we've discussed, secretion of melatonin decreases with passing years as the pineal gland ages and becomes calcified. Very old people make almost none, compared with levels secreted by young people. Have you ever been amazed at how a small child can sleep through anything? That's the wisdom of the child's growing body, giving itself plenty of deep sleep to allow growth of bones, muscles, and organs. It accomplishes this by pumping out a hefty dose of melatonin. During sleep, surges of growth hormone radiate throughout the body, stimulating the growth of healthy tissues.

Scientists have speculated that the pineal gland may in fact be the "aging clock" that causes us to age and die within the appropriate span of years. These researchers reason that with the replacement of the pineal hormone melatonin, this aging clock can be set back dramatically.

In 1994, researchers discovered that melatonin induces sleep. It then became widely available as a supplement. Continued research revealed that melatonin plays a role in immunity and sexual health, and that it is a very powerful neutralizer of free radicals.

The youth-preserving potential of melatonin has been illustrated vividly in studies of mice: those given melatonin lived months longer (the equivalent of years in a human) and enjoyed robust good health right up until their death. Strains of mice susceptible to cancer succumbed to the disease significantly less often, and later in life, when given melatonin. Mice given melatonin have shiny, thick coats into old age, while those not given the hormone end up with dull, patchy coats. Because mice are nocturnal and melatonin therefore works differently in them, we don't know how much of this research can be extrapolated to humans, but it's tantalizing just the same.

There has been some controversy as to whether melatonin should be made available only by prescription. Those who oppose the over-the-counter sale of melatonin warn that the supplements are not regulated and could be contaminated; they warn that large doses of hormones can be dangerous; and they warn that the long-term effects of supplementation in humans are unknown. In his book *Melatonin: Nature's Sleeping Pill,* Ray Sahelian, M.D., makes some astute observations about the motives of those who would make melatonin a prescription drug, stating that "even medicines approved by the FDA have in some cases been found to be contaminated, or have serious health risks. The food we eat can be contaminated. . . . Why raise the contamination issue expressly with melatonin and unnecessarily alarm the public?" He also says that any medicine, in excess, has the potential to be dangerous. The motives of those who are pushing for melatonin to be regulated as a prescription drug may be driven less by a concern for public safety than by the potential for financial gain: If this hormone is as potent a sleep aid, disease preventive, and youth preserver as it appears to be in the research done thus far, there are millions upon millions of dollars to be made on the patent and sale of melatonin by pharmaceutical companies.

Sleep allows the body to focus its energy on healing and restoration, and when an aging pineal gland doesn't make adequate quantities of melatonin, sleep duration and quality both suffer. A dose of 1 to 3 milligrams of melatonin taken a half-hour before bed soothes the body into a deep sleep that is interrupted less often. One of the major complaints I hear from people with insomnia is that lack of sleep at night leads to mental fuzziness and physical exhaustion the next day.

They never feel that they've gotten enough rest. With plenty of sound, rejuvenating sleep, the body is able to function better during waking hours.

For shift workers or frequent travelers, melatonin is a great tool for resetting the body's sleep-wake clock. All you need to do is take it a half-hour before bedtime. Unlike prescription sleeping pills, melatonin has no known side effects and won't cause drowsiness the following day unless you take large amounts.

As far as the exciting potential of melatonin as an anti-aging, cancer-fighting, and antioxidant supplement goes, it's important to remember that most of the research that's been done so far has been on rodents and in test tubes or petri dishes *(in vitro)*. The effect of melatonin on mice is spectacular, but remember that mice don't make melatonin in their bodies. Therefore, to project the effectiveness of melatonin on mice onto humans is a giant leap of faith; further study is needed.

This is not to say that if a man is middle-aged or older he shouldn't try melatonin, or even use it regularly as a sleep aid or anti-aging supplement. The research so far is exciting.

Here are some guidelines for sufferers of insomnia and their partners:

- Make sure the bed is used only for sleeping and spending quality time together.
- Don't read, talk on the phone, work, or watch television in bed.
- Condition your body to know that the bed is a place for sleeping.
- Don't drink caffeinated beverages or eat chocolate after 3 P.M.
- Don't exercise within two or three hours of bedtime, but do exercise—it will enhance the quality of sleep to have had a good workout that day.
- If stress is keeping you awake, try some meditation or relaxed deep breathing before bed.

- A high-complex-carbohydrate snack induces sleepiness by causing the release of tryptophan, melatonin's precursor amino acid.
- Calcium/magnesium supplements or the herb valerian are other sleep aids to try.
- If you want to try melatonin, take 1 to 3 milligrams a half-hour to an hour before bed no more than three times a week. The sublingual variety, which you dissolve under your tongue, is absorbed more rapidly, so you may want to take that closer to bedtime than you would the tablets.

5

Keeping Cells Young by Squelching Oxidation

My patient George is a sun-worshipper who has maintained his deep golden tan for decades. Now that he's in his fifties, all those years in the sun are beginning to take their toll. His face and neck are much more deeply lined than they should be for someone his age, and dark spots have sprung up on his face and hands. He's started to be more careful, but at his initial examination I discovered a cancerous mole on his shoulder. Luckily, we caught it early and he'll be fine.

Matthew is a traveling salesman who looks considerably older than his forty-seven years. His diet while on the road consists mainly of fast-food takeout, airline food, and packaged cakes and cookies. "I just don't have time to think about what I eat," he tells me during our consultation. "Besides, I've been reading about this new weight loss diet that lets you eat as much fat and protein as you want, even red meat. So having a fast-food cheeseburger and a candy bar might be just what the doctor ordered." Gently, I tell him that if the results of lab tests of his cholesterol, blood sugars, and hormones are any indication of the healthfulness of his diet, this doctor would not be ordering anything of the sort for him.

Dave, another patient of mine, finally kicked a twenty-five-year smoking habit after a bout of chest pains that landed him in the hospital. In his sixties, he consulted me soon after he had been told by another physician that without triple bypass surgery he would soon die. "I picked up a few of those books about chelation therapy and using vitamins and diet changes to cure heart disease," he tells me during his first visit. "Smoking's supposed to make you a lot more likely to have heart troubles, too, so I finally quit. It makes sense to try these kinds of things first, before I let them crack my ribcage open and stop my heart, right?" I have to agree with him on that point.

What George, Matthew, and Dave have in common is that they all have been exposed to something that has dramatically increased the level of *oxidative stress* their bodies experience. Increased oxidation means increased production of *free radicals,* which in turn means increased risk of skin degeneration, cancer, and heart disease. Sunlight, toxins such as food additives and preservatives, and cigarettes all wreak their havoc within the body this way.

WHAT IS OXIDATION?

The very first creatures that inhabited this planet didn't breathe oxygen; in fact, they died if exposed to too high a concentration of this gas we now depend on for life. Oxygen spurred oxidation in these primitive life forms, producing unstable molecules known as free radicals. Free radicals could quickly cause the demise of these creatures.

The evolution and spread of plants, which produce oxygen during photosynthesis, has created an atmosphere over our planet's surface that is 21 percent oxygen. This, in turn, has brought about the evolution of *aerobic* animals whose bodies are specifically equipped to use oxygen, and *antioxidant* systems to combat its damaging by-products, the free radicals.

Food isn't a totally clean-burning fuel; it leaves waste and free radicals behind, similar to a car's exhaust after burning gasoline. Your body makes free radicals as it breaks down the food you eat and turns it into energy. Every moment of your life, your cells are breaking down fuel in order to stay alive and perform their functions in your body. Oxygen, brought to all the cells via the blood vessels, plays an important role in this process, which is why we can't live without it.

Biological warfare is going on at this very moment throughout your body. As free radicals are created by oxidation reactions, the antioxidants engage in a valiant struggle to neutralize these toxic particles before they can do too much damage. Oxidation reactions happen millions of times a second in your body, but you have a very sophisticated array of antioxidant defenses to deal with them.

ANTIOXIDANTS: YOUR BODY'S DEFENSE AGAINST FREE RADICALS

When we are young and healthy and taking good care of ourselves, there's a balance between formation of free radicals and antioxidant defenses. The rate at which the body pumps out free radicals increases during times of stress. Hard exercise, being sick, suffering an injury, or just feeling "stressed out" all have this effect. Excessive exposure to toxins such as cigarette smoke, car exhaust, pesticides, solvents, and radiation also accelerates free radical production.

The antioxidant defenses can rise to the challenge to a point, but too much oxidation can become overwhelming. Free radicals spill over and start deadly chain reactions that destroy cells. The common thread that connects nearly all the diseases that afflict aging people is thought to be this imbalance between free radicals created by oxidation reactions and the antioxidants that neutralize them.

Free radicals aren't all bad. They do have some important functions in the body. They act as messengers between cells, play a part in enzyme reactions, and are used by the immune system as weapons against invading bacteria and viruses. For this reason, we don't want to go overboard with the antioxidants and take megadoses. Once again, with experimentation your partner will find the dose that's right for his body.

INFLAMMATION AND OXIDATION: YOU CAN'T HAVE ONE WITHOUT THE OTHER

When you twist your ankle, it may become swollen, hot, and red. If so, you have experienced an *inflammatory response,* in which the immune system sends dozens of different kinds of cells and extra fluid to the injured part. Dead cells and bacteria are removed with the excess fluid as new cells grow to heal the injury.

Where there is inflammation, there are free radicals; and when there is already an imbalance between free radicals and antioxidants, it can exacerbate the inflammatory response. The rising incidence of autoimmune diseases like rheumatoid arthritis, lupus, and allergies is due in part to out-of-control inflammation. Supplemental antioxidants and essential fatty acids can help you control inflammation without resorting to prescription drugs. Refer to the section at the end of this chapter for guidelines.

THE CHAIN REACTION OF OXIDATION

If you sprinkle lemon juice on sliced apples, you are adding vitamin C, an antioxidant, to the exposed white center of the apple and stopping the oxidative process that turns it brown.

Oxidation reactions occur when oxygen reacts with something in the body or the environment that creates unstable molecules called free radicals. Free radicals ricochet around, looking for something to latch onto, but unless they latch onto an antioxidant, they'll make whatever they latch onto unstable, and start a chain reaction.

For example, a free radical that encounters an unsaturated fat in the bloodstream will latch onto it and oxidize it, turning it rancid. Rancid fats have been implicated as an important cause of blood vessel disease, which can lead to heart attacks and strokes.

If free radicals latch onto DNA, the cells' genetic coding system, they can throw the cells' production of essential proteins out of kilter, eventually killing the cells—or, in the worst-case scenario, causing them to become cancerous.

YOUR ANTIOXIDANT ARSENAL

Antioxidants have the important job of protecting you from free radical damage. The body can manufacture some of these antioxidants with the right raw materials. Glutathione, melatonin, and coenzyme Q10 are some examples of these *endogenous* antioxidants that are manufactured in the body. Others, like the vitamins A, C, and E, and the mineral selenium, have to be taken in as part of the foods one eats. These are known as essential vitamins and minerals.

The antioxidants renew each other once they are spent; for example, vitamin E that has neutralized a free radical is "recharged" by vitamin C. Glutathione is recharged by beta carotene, vitamin C, and vitamin E. Without all the antioxidants present, those that are oxidized in the process of buffering free radicals may not be neutralized themselves and can cause cellular damage. That's why it's a good idea to take an antioxidant supplement that contains all the nutrients that cooperate with one another to battle the free radical onslaught your body faces every day. I'll give you guidelines for picking antioxidant supplements near the end of this chapter.

Our world is filled with toxins, our stress levels are high, and we tend to eat processed foods stripped of their nutrients. In other words, our bodies are being asked to handle a much larger free radical load with reduced defenses! It's no wonder that degenerative diseases are on the rise. The more help a man can give his body in the struggle to keep oxidation from overwhelming it, the more years of health he's likely to enjoy.

In recent years we have just begun to appreciate the amazing power of the antioxidants made in the body. Glutathione, ubiquinone (more commonly referred to as coenzyme Q10), catalase, superoxide dismutase (SOD), melatonin, and alpha lipoic acid are some of the body's built-in antioxidant defenses; some are available in supplement form.

GLUTATHIONE: THE MASTER ANTIOXIDANT

Glutathione is an amino acid manufactured in the liver in humans and is found in every cell of every plant and animal. When you're in good health you produce about 14,000 milligrams (14 grams) per day—that's eight and a half tablespoons! This important antioxidant is amazingly adept at squelching free radical chain reactions. Glutathione levels in ill people are almost always low. That's because the body uses much of its supply to fight off the oxidative damage done by disease.

Glutathione is too large a molecule to be digested, and it's very unstable, so it isn't available in supplement form. You can raise your glutathione levels by eating foods rich in sulfur, because sulfur is needed to build this essential antioxidant. Sulfur is found in eggs, garlic, onions, and asparagus, for example. Both MSM (methylsulfonylmethane) and alpha-lipoic acid are sulfur-rich antioxidant compounds made in your body. Alpha-lipoic acid also directly supports liver detoxification. Supplementing with these nutrients is a good way to enhance your body's production of glutathione. With the MSM, the dosage is 500 milligrams 1 to 3 times daily, and the dosage for alpha-lipoic acid is 500 milligrams per day in divided doses. Use caution with alpha-lipoic acid if you have diabetes—it can cause blood sugar to dip.

The amino acid *cysteine* is another component of glutathione, and N-acetyl-cysteine (NAC) can be used as a dietary supplement to raise glutathione levels. Try 500 milligrams 2 to 3 times a day.

The vitamins *beta-carotene, C,* and *E* and the mineral *selenium,* all antioxidants in their own right, have additional roles as reenergizers of glutathione. I'll tell you how much of these to take later in this chapter.

Milk thistle *(silymarin)* is an herb that boosts glutathione levels in the liver. The liver is where your body processes toxins, so it's especially important to keep antioxidant defenses strong there. Take 120 milligrams or the equivalent 3 times a day.

MELATONIN

The pineal gland, a tiny endocrine organ nestled in the brain, is triggered to release melatonin into the bloodstream when darkness falls. Only 125 trillionths of a gram puts you to sleep for the night. Your body's ability to make adequate amounts of melatonin is impaired as you age, which is why older people often have trouble falling asleep and staying asleep. In very aged people the nighttime rise in melatonin levels is barely perceptible. The deep sleep that allows the body to renew itself becomes a thing of the past. (Refer to chapter 4 for more about melatonin as a sleep aid.)

Researchers are discovering that melatonin has many other functions in the body as well, including that of a very effective free radical scavenger. It's especially good at protecting DNA from free radical attack. Melatonin also works to promote the action of glutathione. Some speculate that the pineal gland may be the body's "aging clock," with declining secretion of melatonin at the root of the body's decline with passing years.

Melatonin supplements are available in health-food stores. See page 214 for supplementation guidelines.

COENZYME Q10

The *mitochondria* are the "engine" of the cell, where the complex chain reaction that converts glucose molecules to energy takes place. Coenzyme Q10—also called *ubiquinone* (from the word *ubiquitous,* meaning present everywhere at the same time), because it is found naturally in the cells of all life forms—is a crucial part of that chain reaction. Without it, the cell can't produce the energy it needs to perform all its functions and will eventually die. Concentrations of CoQ10 are high in organs and systems that require a lot of energy, such as the heart, liver, and immune system. Recent research is showing that CoQ10 may play an important role in the reactivation and stabilization of vitamin C in the body.

You might have already guessed that aging diminishes the body's ability to make sufficient CoQ10, and that levels tend to be low in those with diseases of aging.

The heart is especially vulnerable to free radical damage. The arteries that feed its walls can become clogged with oxidized fats, blocking the flow of oxygen-rich blood to the heart muscle. Coenzyme Q10 is made in your body and has been shown to energize the heart's pumping action in addition to squelching free radicals. It has been shown to be useful in the treatment of high blood pressure as well.

When researchers found that concentrations of CoQ10 were very low in the gum tissues of those with severe gum disease, they tried giving patients supplemental CoQ10. The results were incredible, with complete reversal of even the most serious cases.

Positive effects on the immune system, athletic performance, and obesity have also been shown in studies involving CoQ10. With all this evidence of benefit and no risk at appropriate doses, it's a sure bet for inclusion in a youth-preserving, free radical–buffering supplement plan. Try supplementing anywhere from 30 to 200 milligrams per day.

VITAMIN C

The evidence to support the use of large doses of vitamin C for health and longevity is overwhelming. The work of Linus Pauling and Ewan Cameron convincingly showed how supplementation of vitamin C could fight off the common cold, heart disease, and cancer. It's truly remarkable to me that supplemental use of vitamin C is not universal. If there were a drug this effective on the market, advertising would be splattered on every billboard across the country.

Aside from its duties as a free radical scavenger, vitamin C is a potent immune system booster that gives your body a great deal more power for fighting off illness. It is also an element of collagen, the material that binds cells together. Vitamin C deficiency causes skin, mucous membranes, and blood vessels to weaken.

Our need for vitamin C increases when we are sick or under a lot of stress. Very ill people can take up to 17,000 milligrams (17 grams) per day, and their bodies will use it all. The U.S. Recommended Daily Allowance (RDA) is only 60 milligrams. I recommend at least 2,000 milligrams per day when you're healthy, and three to five times that when you're sick. Take it in divided doses, and if its acidity upsets your stomach, try a buffered form or reduce the dose. Eat citrus fruits, mangoes, kiwi, red peppers, potatoes, and tomatoes, all of which are rich in vitamin C.

VITAMIN E

This fat-soluble antioxidant has been thoroughly researched as an adjunct to medical therapy for heart disease. It is especially good for preventing the oxidation of cholesterol and fats in the bloodstream, and protects the B vitamins, red blood cells, and hormones from being oxidized by free radicals. It can reenergize both vitamins C and A after they do their antioxidant work.

Vitamin E plays a pivotal role in the muscle and heart cells, helping to provide them with a continuous supply of fuel. It's a mild blood thinner that staves off the formation of tiny blood clots that can clog blood vessels. Wheat germ, whole grains, and nuts are good food sources, but it's a good idea to supplement your dietary intake with 400 IU (international units) daily of vitamin E derived from alpha-tocopherol.

BETA-CAROTENE, VITAMIN A, AND THE CAROTENOIDS

Beta-carotene works alongside vitamin E as a free radical scavenger, and is needed for maintenance and growth of the mucous membranes of the nose, throat, and lungs. One-quarter to one-half of the beta-carotene you eat is converted into vitamin A. Your eyes need this fat-soluble vitamin to make the pigments that give us night vision. Preformed vitamin A can be toxic in large doses, but it's safe to take 10,000 to 15,000 IU of beta-carotene per day, and up to 10,000 IU of preformed vitamin A daily.

Lycopene, lutein, and zeaxanthin are other carotenoids that effectively fight free radical damage. Leafy green vegetables are excellent sources of these nutrients. Try to eat spinach, kale, collard, or other greens four or five times a week.

SELENIUM

This trace element has recently caused a stir in research circles because of its powerful antioxidant properties. It works with vitamin E to keep fats from being oxidized in the bloodstream. Selenium is thought to play a role in cellular energy production, and is needed to make glutathione and *prostaglandins,* which help regulate blood pressure and inflammation. Researchers are well on their way to proving that selenium can help prevent many types of cancer. I recommend 200 micrograms per day, either in a multivitamin or as an individual supplement. During a viral infection such as the flu or a herpes outbreak, the dose can be as much as 1,000 micrograms (1 milligram) daily for a week.

REDUCING YOUR OXIDATIVE LOAD

At the other end of the equation of reducing free radicals, there's lessening the body's oxidative load. This can be accomplished by eating a healthy diet low in pesticides and preservatives, avoiding toxins such as car exhaust and fumes from solvents such as acetone, managing the stress in life (attitude is everything here!), nipping illnesses in the bud whenever possible, and not engaging in overly strenuous exercise too often.

A MULTIVITAMIN A DAY KEEPS THE DOCTOR AWAY

I recommend that everyone invest in a high-potency multivitamin to complement a healthy diet and use of anti-aging supplements. The two-a-day variety is best; one-a-day multivitamins don't keep levels of life-giving nutrients as consistently high as do those taken throughout the day. Take one with breakfast or lunch and one with dinner, so that the nutrients can be absorbed with food. Choose a multivitamin that includes the following nutrients:

- Beta-carotene/carotenoids: 10,000 to 15,000 IU
- Vitamin A: 5,000 to 10,000 IU

- The B vitamins:
    Thiamine (B$_1$): 25 to 50 milligrams
    Riboflavin (B$_2$): 25 to 100 milligrams
    Niacin (B$_3$): 50 to 100 milligrams
    Pantothenic acid (B$_5$): 50 to 100 milligrams
    Pyridoxine (B$_6$): 50 to 100 milligrams
    Vitamin B$_{12}$: 1,000 to 2,000 micrograms
    Biotin: 100 to 300 micrograms
    Choline: 50 to 100 milligrams
    Folic acid (folate or folacin): 400 to 800 micrograms
- Inositol: 150 to 300 milligrams
- Calcium: 300 to 500 milligrams for men, 600 to 800 milligrams for women
- Vitamin D: 100 to 400 IU
- Vitamin C: 2,000 to 10,000 milligrams
- Vitamin E: 400 IU
- Boron: 1 to 5 milligrams
- Chromium: 200 to 400 micrograms
- Copper: 1 to 5 milligrams
- Magnesium: 300 to 500 milligrams
- Manganese: 5 to 10 milligrams
- Selenium: 200 micrograms
- Vanadyl sulfate: 5 to 10 milligrams
- Zinc: 10 to 15 milligrams

Notice the absence of iron in this recommendation? Men should choose a multivitamin without iron, unless they have been diagnosed with anemia. With the recent discoveries about free radicals causing many degenerative diseases, iron has been researched for its potential as a catalyst for the oxidation process. Too much iron in the bloodstream has been linked to heart disease and some kinds of cancer. Too much iron can overwhelm the body's antioxidant defenses. My dietary recommendations provide plenty of iron. Iron toxicity is another reason to limit processed baked goods, cereals, and pastas: these products are generously enriched with iron. Very few men are deficient in iron, in contrast to teenage girls and premenopausal women, in whom iron deficiency is more common because of monthly loss of blood during menstruation.

A DAILY ANTIOXIDANT SUPPLEMENT IS GOOD HEALTH INSURANCE

Because it's impossible to pack all the nutrients necessary for optimal health into one or two tablets, it's best to take extra vitamin C (enough to total at least 2,000 milligrams per day) and beta-carotene (enough to total 15 to 25,000 IU per day), and make sure they're combined with a few bioflavonoid antioxidants such as grapeseed extract, green tea, or quercetin. Many excellent antioxidant supplements are available. Take them whenever you take the multivitamin. During illness, stress, or heavy workouts, or when there is inflammation from an injury, illness, or an allergy, extra doses of antioxidants throughout the day are a good idea. You can double or triple your dose.

You may be shaking your head and saying to yourself, "He won't want to take all these vitamins every day—two multivitamins, plus extra antioxidants and all the other stuff—it's too much trouble!" I know it's a difficult adjustment to make. I recommend buying one of those pill-dose boxes at the drugstore, filling it with all the vitamins needed for the day, with separate compartments for each mealtime, and carrying the box with you. Taking a handful of supplements every day is an inconvenience only when you forget the long-term benefits.

6

Maintaining Muscle for Life

"With only five minutes a day, once a week, the Abdomenicizer can transform you from your pitiful, potbellied present self to a rippled Adonis! It can be yours now for only three easy payments of $29.95 plus $25 shipping and handling. Act now while supplies last!"

"The breakthrough Cream Cheese and Garlic Diet plus our exclusive Heat-Preserving, Cellulite-Reducing Body Wraps have worked miracles for Joe, Helen, and Jason. Let's talk to them now. . . ."

"Wanna know how I got this body? The E-Z Toner! It whittles, tightens, tones, and burns 1,500 calories an hour without the harmful impact of walking or joint stress of lifting weights. Best of all, it fits right in your walk-in closet! Take advantage of our special offer and call now with a major credit card. . . ."

Okay, maybe I'm exaggerating a little, but you've seen and heard for yourselves the advertisements and infomercials featuring self-proclaimed fitness gurus hawking the latest miracle cream, machine, or diet.

The average person doesn't know enough about how the body works to know how to sift the wheat from the chaff when bombarded by all of this misinformation. You may already have purchased one of those fitness gadgets, and it's probably collecting dust now because it didn't do what the buff guy in the tight polo shirt promised.

Some guys never seem to have to worry about their bodies. They are the ones who hike and bike and walk nearly every day, or the recreational athletes who devote lots of time and energy to their sport. Staying fit is part of their lifestyle.

At the other extreme are the guys who sit at desks all day long and sit in their cars or on their couches the rest of the time. At the end of a long day of work, exercise is the last thing they want to do. Occasionally they manage to motivate themselves to buy a gym membership, a video, or a piece of equipment to use at home. Once the initial push is over, though, they lose steam fast, and they're back to their old sedentary ways.

At first glance, you might not be able to tell the difference between a twenty-five-year-old active person and a sedentary person of the same age. It's the slow but persistent passage of time that brings out the visible differences. Creeping weight gain and deterioration of muscle and bone happen much earlier in life and to a greater extent in people who don't exercise.

If the man in your life falls into the first category described above, he's already doing a lot to maintain his health and help himself weather andropause. This chapter should give him (and you) some extra encouragement and up-to-date information.

If he falls into the latter category, don't despair—it's never too late to start building muscle and conditioning the cardiovascular system. In this chapter I'm going to give you all the tools he needs to get started. I'm also going to make sure you and he know how to get the most benefit in the least amount of time.

USE IT OR LOSE IT

The body is a marvelously efficient piece of machinery. It's constantly seeking out ways to survive with as little effort as possible. A body part that isn't used for some time tends to weaken, shrink, or even disappear, and the energy once used for the maintenance of that body part is redirected. That's where the expression "use it or lose it" comes from.

Muscle uses a lot of energy, and the body's wisdom reasons that if it can pare down the muscle, energy requirements will be lower—which is desirable when food is scarce. Fat, on the other hand, requires almost no energy for maintenance, and the body can accrue large amounts of it. For people living with the threat of starvation, this is a good thing, but in our culture of plenty, fat is not a good thing.

The body will adapt to whatever level of activity we give it. If we don't get any exercise, the body perceives no necessity to maintain the muscle mass needed to do that activity. Excess calories taken in are then stored as fat. Storing fat as energy is a very efficient process, but building and maintaining muscle tissue is relatively less so. In the name of efficiency, the body will preferentially store excess calories taken in as fat—unless we exercise.

Exercise sends a message throughout the body that it needs to devote resources to the maintenance of muscle tissue and to keeping the heart and lungs in good function. The unprecedented level of physical ease in our lives has made it necessary to willfully impose stress, in the form of exercise, on our bodies to stay fit. This is especially true as we grow older.

Essentially, exercise is about decreasing the body's efficiency: trying to make more work, burn more calories, and use more energy.

WHY THE BODY SUCCUMBS TO THE PULL OF GRAVITY

Let's look at the example of a man who enjoys lots of time on the couch with a bag of greasy chips, and who thinks exercise is something you do once a week in a game of pickup basketball. By the time he celebrates his seventieth birthday, he can expect to have lost 30 percent of lean mass (including muscle, bone, and organs) and to have increased the amount of fat he's lugging around by 50 percent. That doesn't necessarily mean he'll weigh more—fat weighs about half as much as muscle—but it does mean his clothes won't fit, he'll have a "spare tire," his strength and endurance will not be what they once were, and he certainly won't want to be on the team that goes shirtless when they play basketball. After the age of forty, the muscles and organs begin to shrink, and bones become porous and weakened as minerals are lost over the years.

The good news is that we can greatly modulate the assault of time on the body. Some wear and tear is inevitable, of course, but we can do a lot to slow it down. A physically fit septuagenarian can run a sedentary thirty-year-old into the ground.

Preserving muscle is an important part of preserving youth. Exercise, particularly resistance training, is a key component of a muscle-maintaining regimen. Not only does muscle look good, but a properly conditioned, resistance-trained body functions better than one that isn't—it's more flexible, more virile, and accomplishes everyday tasks with much greater ease. The right nutritional supplements can also help give the body what it needs to keep muscles powerful.

Declining levels of muscle-building hormones such as growth hormone and testosterone are largely to blame for "middle-age spread." In chapters 4 and 5, you read about these hormones, and later in this chapter I'll give you some specific protocols for muscle-building hormone replacement.

Hormonal decline is not the only culprit, though. As people age they tend to be less active, and this decrease in activity has a significant effect on how fast we age. No one seems to know for sure how much influence this trend has on the fattening of Americans, but it certainly isn't helping us in our quest to stay slim.

GETTING YOUR HEART MUSCLE IN SHAPE

Walking, cycling, jogging, hiking, stairclimbing, and other kinds of cardiovascular exercise get the heart beating faster, the lungs working harder, and the circulation pumping better. The focus of most of the rest of this chapter is going to be on muscle-building exercise, but I also want to stress the importance of getting five to seven aerobic workouts a week.

The latest guidelines say that any activity that involves getting off the chair and moving around is enough to have a positive influence on our health. This is absolutely true for sedentary people: thirty minutes of gentle walking a day can be the bridge from inactivity to activity. Then, doing more physical activity will yield even greater benefits.

At the other end of the continuum, too much or too intense exercise is counterproductive, diminishing immune function and causing a dramatic increase in free radical production. It's important that competitive athletes or anyone who simply prefers hard, long aerobic workouts take especially good care of themselves by taking lots of antioxidants, eating well, and getting plenty of rest.

ABOUT TARGET HEART RATE

Say he's finally gotten off the couch and out the door. It's a gorgeous, crisp fall day, and he breaks into a brisk walk. It feels so good, he wonders what he's been waiting for all these years. As he rounds the corner and starts up a hill, his breath gets shorter, and he feels his heart beginning to pound. By the time he reaches the top, he realizes just how out of shape he is. With each new day, he walks a little farther or a little faster. In a month's time, he can stride up that hill that was once so forbidding without even feeling out of breath, and his heart beats strong, steady, and slow as he climbs.

What's happened? On the very first day of his walking program, his cardiovascular system was under serious stress. The unaccustomed work of exercising placed a demand on the heart and lungs to send extra oxygen to the muscles. If this demand is repeatedly placed on the body—that is, if we continue to exercise day after day—the body responds by making the heart muscle stronger, the lungs more efficient, and the vessels throughout the body more open to the flow of blood. With each beat, the aerobically fit heart can pump more blood than the unfit one. The heart rate of an elite endurance athlete at rest can be as low as forty beats per minute—about half of the average person's resting heart rate! Suggest that he try counting his heart rate for a full minute just as he awakens in the morning, when he's totally relaxed. Write that number down. After a month of regular cardiovascular exercise, check it again and see how much it's gone down. That's the heart increasing its pumping power!

Measuring heart rate during exercise is a reasonably good way to gauge how hard he's working, and can show how his cardiovascular fitness is improving. As he gets fitter, his heart gets stronger and can do more work with less effort, so it doesn't have to pump as fast to keep him going through a workout. When the heart rate doesn't climb as high as it did when he last did some aerobic exercise, it's time to pick up the speed, find a route with more hills, or otherwise increase the intensity of his chosen mode of exercise. His body then will be challenged further and he will become even fitter.

Use this formula to calculate the target heart rate range:

1. 220 minus his age = the age-predicted maximum heart rate. (If he is fifty years old, his predicted maximum is around 170 beats per minute.)

2. Multiply his maximum heart rate by 65 percent (0.65) and 85 percent (0.85).

The low number is the bottom of his target range, and the high number is at the top. Divide these numbers by 6 to get an easy 10 second count, so that he can take his pulse more quickly.

You've probably seen people running and cycling while wearing heart rate monitors that strap around the ribcage and send a signal to a watch that gives you a readout of your heart rate in beats per minute. These monitors give a pretty accurate reading, which can be hard to do ourselves as we tear along on the Stairmaster at breakneck speed. A pulse monitor will measure in beats per minute.

If a man is taking beta-blockers or other drugs to treat high blood pressure or an irregular heartbeat, his heart rate may not accurately reflect how hard he's exercising. He must pay attention instead to how he's feeling as he works out—the ideal is to be a little out of breath and sweaty, but still be able to hold a conversation. If he is taking any prescription drugs, especially those for high blood pressure, diabetes, or heart disease, he must be sure to consult his doctor before he starts any exercise program.

LOSE THE FAT, KEEP THE MUSCLE

It isn't possible to spot-reduce the belly or the thighs with ab crunches or leg lifts. Strengthening exercises can build muscle, but it won't show if it's beneath a layer of fat. Simultaneously building muscle and losing excess body fat will let those washboard abs show through.

Increasing energy expenditure through exercise and decreasing food intake is the way to rid ourselves of excess body fat. There's even an "afterburn" effect that keeps the metabolism slightly elevated for a few hours after exercise.

Moderate cardiovascular exercise (in his target heart rate range) puts the body into fat-burning mode. To supply the needed energy for a run or brisk walk, the body delves into fat stores and breaks them down. By getting into better cardiovascular condition, the body can access fat stores earlier in a workout, so that fat-burning ability increases.

When we do moderate to intense aerobic exercise (70 to 85 percent of maximum heart rate), the pituitary gland is stimulated to pump out more growth hormone. Elevated growth hormone levels can be maintained into old age with regular cardiovascular and strength training exercise, and that means preservation of lean muscle and loss of excess fat.

FREQUENCY, INTENSITY, AND DURATION

To put together a cardiovascular exercise regimen that works, it's helpful to break it down into three components:

Frequency: the number of times per week
Intensity: how hard to work
Duration: the length of each cardiovascular workout

Let's assume a man has a limited amount of spare time to work out, and can only get to the gym three times a week for thirty minutes each time. This requires cramming cardiovascular and resistance training into that half-hour. A good approach might be to do three short, high-intensity cardiovascular workouts a week, getting the heart rate up to the top of the target range for fifteen to twenty minutes, and then doing a circuit of a couple of sets each of weight-training exercises. When the frequency and duration are low, the intensity should be higher.

A man who has more time but doesn't feel like joining a gym can settle into a walking routine, perhaps a four-mile loop each morning at a fairly brisk pace, sending the heart rate up to 65 or 70 percent of maximum. He can lift weights or take yoga classes three or four times a week. When the frequency and duration are high, the intensity can be low.

It is important for any man to tailor his workouts to his own preferences and schedule. Keep in mind, though, that the more intense a workout he can handle, the more the growth hormone levels rise, and the more calories he'll expend.

WORKOUTS THAT BUILD MUSCLE

Weight training doesn't have to mean straining to bench-press his own body weight or doing straight-legged deadlifts until his intervertebral disks burst. It is, however, hard work, and physically demanding on the body. The whole point of resistance training is to fool the body into thinking it needs to make more muscle, bone, and connective tissue to do all the hard lifting and carrying required of it.

The science of weight training is complicated, but a few basics should clarify it.

THE IMPORTANCE OF PROPER ALIGNMENT

Suggest to your man that he stand in front of a full-length mirror and together look at his posture. First, have him stand so that he can see himself from the side. Are his shoulders slumped? Is his neck perpendicular to the floor, or is it jutting forward? Is his chest thrust forward, shoulders tightly pinched up and back?

Now look at his hips and his trunk. Is his pelvis thrust forward so that he looks as though he were born without a butt? Does he have the gentle indentation in his lower back known as the lumbar curve? If the curve is there, is it extremely pronounced?

Now have him face the mirror. Is one shoulder higher than the other? Are the hips even? Look at his feet. Is his weight evenly distributed along the heel, ball, and toes, or does he stand on the outside or inside edges of his feet?

Proper posture means using the body in the way it's made to be used, according to the biomechanical principles of its design. Watch a toddler pick something up from the ground—you'll notice that rather than bending at the waist, he'll squat, keeping his torso erect. Years of slouching in uncomfortable chairs for hours at a time, coupled with lack of exercise and body awareness, train us out of those natural movement patterns and into bad habits like locking our knees and bending at the waist to pick up large items.

If proper alignment is important in everyday life, it's doubly important in resistance training, which dramatically increases the loads the joints have to carry.

Many workout programs and body healing techniques such as the Alexander technique, Feldenkrais, chi kung, and yoga classes will help improve posture.

WEIGHT TRAINING BASICS

Once a man is aware of the need for proper body alignment and has something to achieve, he can decide on the type of workout. If he'd rather work out at home than at a gym, he can do so without much expense. A bench and three sets of dumbbells—5, 10, and 15 pounds—should be adequate to start. If he does decide to join a gym, be sure he sets up an appointment with a trainer to acclimate him to the equipment. It might be costly, but it's worth it to have the instruction. Even if he decides he'd rather work out at home, it should be easy enough to find a certified personal trainer to get him started safely.

A comprehensive resistance training program should include exercises for the shoulders, back, arms, abdominals, and legs. Three nonconsecutive days a week (e.g., Monday, Wednesday, and Friday; or Tuesday, Thursday, and Saturday) are best if the goal is to build muscle, and a minimum of two workouts a week is necessary for maintenance of lean mass.

He should do one to three sets of ten to fifteen repetitions of each exercise. He should perform the exercises slowly, taking a slow count of two for the first half (the lifting of the weight against gravity—the *concentric,* or shortening, contraction) and a slow count of three for the second (the lowering of the weight back toward gravity—the *eccentric,* or lengthening, contraction). He should breathe in deeply during the concentric phase and out during the eccentric phase.

Each set should be done to fatigue, which means he couldn't manage another repetition without cheating. What is the correct amount of weight to lift? He should be able to do eight to fifteen reps before the muscles are fatigued. Make sure he rests for at least thirty seconds between sets. Once he can perform three sets of an exercise without feeling fatigued, the weight should be increased at the next workout. He should start out with one or two sets at the new weight and work up to doing more.

There are literally thousands of weight-training exercises he can do. I recommend Bill Pearl and Gary T. Moran's classic book, *Getting Stronger,* as a comprehensive guide to the possibilities.

Any man with back, knee, or shoulder problems must be extremely cautious when beginning a weight training program. Reinjury is a real danger if he doesn't do the exercise using correct form.

The following seven exercises should get him off to a good start.

Bench Press

Lie on your back on a bench. Place your feet firmly on the ground and slightly tilt your hips up so that your lower back isn't arched. Grasp a 10- or 15-pound dumbbell in each hand, holding the elbows at 90 degrees with the upper arms parallel and the forearms perpendicular to the floor. Pinch your shoulder blades together so that your chest feels opened up, shoulders rolled back. Take a deep inhalation and as you

exhale, extend both arms straight up until the dumbbells clink together over the center of your chest. Your elbows should be straight at
this point. Return slowly to starting position, inhaling.

Bent-Over Rows
This exercise works the latissimus dorsi, the long back muscle that ex-
tends from the back of the shoulder down to the lower spine. Kneel
with the right knee on the bench and the other foot on the floor. Bend
forward and put the right hand down on the bench so that your back
is flat like a table. Hold a 10- to 20-pound dumbbell in the left hand
with the elbow of the left arm turned in. Inhale. On the exhalation,
draw the left elbow up past your waist. Inhale as you return to starting position.

Shoulder Press
Hold a 5- or 10-pound dumbbell in each hand. You can either sit or
stand. Start with the arms out at right angles, upper arms parallel to
the floor, forearms perpendicular to the floor, elbows out to the sides,
palms facing front. Inhale, and with an exhalation press both arms
straight overhead until the weights meet above your head. Inhale as
you return to starting position.

Bicep Curl
With a 10- to 20-pound dumbbell in each hand, stand with the elbows tucked into the sides, palms facing forward. Inhale, and with an
exhalation curl both hands toward the shoulders, taking care to keep
the elbows locked in to the waist. Inhale as you return to starting
position.

Squat
Stand with feet hip-width apart, toes pointing forward. You can place
dumbbells or a barbell on your shoulders, but be sure you've mastered
the form before adding extra weight. Exhale as you squat down, and
imagine you're trying to sit in a chair that's several feet behind you.

Your weight should be on your heels, your posterior should be pushing out behind you, your chest should be lifted and expanded, and your gaze should be up. This keeps your back in its natural position with the lumbar curve intact. Take it slow and try to get down to where your thighs are parallel to the floor. Hold there for a moment and inhale as you return to starting position.

Lunges

You may need to hang on to something for balance when you first try this one, but as you get more comfortable you can hold a 10- or 15-pound dumbbell in each hand. Stand with your feet together and take a big step forward with the right foot. There should be about three feet between the front heel and the back toe. Keeping your torso upright, drop the left knee toward the floor, so that the right knee bends to about 90 degrees, with the ankle directly beneath the knee. Push off with the left foot and straighten the right leg to bring the feet back together, and repeat with the other leg, moving across the room. Each lunge is one repetition.

Abdominal Crunch

Lie on your back with knees bent, feet flat on the floor. Use your abdominals to tilt your hips up so that your lower back is pressed down against the floor. Holding that pelvic tilt, place both hands behind your head, gently supporting the head's weight without pulling. Tuck the chin toward the chest and inhale deeply, then raise the top of the shoulders up from the floor by contracting the abdominals. Inhale as you return to the starting position, but don't release all the way down. Repeat 15 to 20 times, rest, and do one or two more sets.

MUSCLE ADAPTATION TO RESISTANCE TRAINING

Resistance training, done properly, actually creates tiny amounts of damage to the muscles. Each muscle is composed of thousands of bundles of muscle fibers. These microscopic fibers contract as one when the muscle is signaled by the nervous system. When the load is more than the muscle is accustomed to bearing, some of the fibers are torn. The repair job creates a fiber that's a bit bigger and stronger than it was.

SUPPLEMENTS FOR MUSCLE POWER

Some supplemental nutrients can help the man who is serious about working out and wants to get the best results he can for his efforts.

Creatine Phosphate

Energy production in the cells boils down to a molecule called adenosine triphosphate (ATP). This molecule is broken apart to generate the energy that makes things happen in the cell. ATP can be renewed faster when there is more available phosphate in the muscles. That's how creatine phosphate helps us to train harder and recover from each set faster—it readily donates its phosphate to ADP (which is "de-energized" ATP) so that it can be broken down again for energy. Harder training and faster recovery means more muscle in less time. For an athlete whose sport requires power and bursts of high-intensity activity, like soccer, basketball, or track and field (throws, sprints, or jumps), creatine should enhance performance. Creatine is found naturally in meats and dairy products; those men who eat mostly vegetarian diets might benefit most from supplementation.

If a man is older than fifty, start with half the following dose and build up. I suggest consulting a nutritionist or athletic trainer about how much to take, and definitely notify your physician that your partner is using creatine.

Buy the powdered form, and have your man start out by taking 15 to 20 grams per day, divided into four doses, for seven days (this is what athletes call a "loading dose"); and then continue with a maintenance dose of 3 to 5 grams per day.

Protein/Branched-Chain Amino Acids

It's a myth that bodybuilders have to eat huge amounts of protein to gain all that mass. The average protein intake of Americans is more than adequate for muscle building, with the exception of very old folks who may not eat enough food. Loading on the protein can actually end up damaging your kidneys. It is interesting to note, though, that meals high in carbohydrates or fats decrease growth hormone secretion, while meals high in protein increase it.

Branched-chain amino acids are components of proteins that have some special characteristics. They can be used as an energy source much more easily than other amino acids, and the results of some studies have caused a lot of excitement among endurance athletes. There isn't much clinical evidence that branched-chains will help build muscle, but a runner or cyclist might try supplementing branched-chains (you can buy the three amino acids—leucine, isoleucine, and valine—as a single supplement at your health-food store). He can expect to feel less tired during his workouts and to recover faster.

Coenzyme Q10

This nutrient is an essential player in the process of cell metabolism. Without it, the cell dies. Supplemental CoQ10 has the effect of enhancing the heart's pumping strength, and there's also some evidence that it can enhance weight loss and muscle repair. Have your man try 30 to 60 milligrams per day.

Chromium

Insulin resistance is the beginning of adult-onset diabetes, and chromium supplements can actually improve the body's uptake of insulin. This means that the body can process carbohydrates more effectively and use them for energy, rather than store them as fat. Your man should take 100 to 200 micrograms per day.

Ginseng

In Chinese medicine, ginseng is what's known as an "adaptogen." Through gentle effects on the endocrine system, adaptogens help the body function better. Ginseng is said to warm the body; boost energy, strength, and endurance; and increase resistance against stress and disease. Studies have shown that people who take Asian ginseng extracts experience increased coordination and alertness. Have your partner try 1 to 2 grams per day; it can be taken in a tea, tincture, or capsule, but make sure the dose is standardized to contain 4 to 7 percent ginsenosides (the active ingredient of the ginseng root). Buy the wild-harvested variety if you can afford it—most cultivated ginseng is heavily sprayed with fungicides.

HORMONES AND MUSCLE BUILDING EXERCISE

Growth Hormone

Exercise is a natural growth hormone booster. As you know from chapter 4, growth hormone has anabolic (tissue-building) and fat-burning effects; and diminishing levels as a man ages results in loss of muscle and gain of fat. Growth hormone supplementation is one way to restore the body we had at twenty-five, but we can do a lot to enhance the body's own production of growth hormone with the right kind of exercise. Moderate to high-intensity aerobic workouts (70 to 90 percent of maximum heart rate) have this effect, and hard resistance training also boosts growth hormone levels. The amino acids arginine, ornithine, lysine, and glutamine are useful growth hormone boosters. Refer to chapter 4 for details on how to supplement these amino acids most effectively. Growth hormone secretion is also stimulated by testosterone.

Testosterone

Testosterone replacement in andropausal men naturally increases muscle size and strength. Testosterone is available only by prescription; see chapter 3 for more information.

Androstenedione

This androgen is transformed to testosterone in the liver. It can be used to increase testosterone levels, which in turn will increase strength and size gains with resistance training. You don't need a prescription to buy androstenedione. Its effects last for about three hours, so the best approach is to take 100 milligrams before weight training. It should not be used more than two or three times a week, because it's not known whether it will dampen the body's own production.

DHEA

Although DHEA supplementation tends to increase testosterone levels in women, it doesn't have the same effect in men. It does slightly raise androstenedione levels, and it may raise estrogen levels. DHEA improves mood and boosts energy, both of which are important for good workouts, and animal studies show an impressive fat-loss effect with supplemental DHEA. If a man is under 50, he can take 2 to 10 milligrams every morning; if he's over 50, he can take 5 to 15 milligrams; if he's over 65, he can take 5 to 25 milligrams.

STRETCHING

Consistent stretching has many benefits; neglecting to stretch sets us up for painful muscle, ligament, and tendon injuries. Stretching exercises should be done after workouts, when the muscles and connective tissues are warm and pliable. Going into the stretch, the goal is to try to reach the very edge of the comfort zone—feeling a pretty powerful pull in the belly of the muscle being stretched—and stay there, breathing deeply and easing further as the muscle lengthens. Don't bounce into a stretch. Hold each one for at least thirty seconds.

There are many books about stretching, but the classics are the ones by Bob Anderson. Easy-to-follow pictures with instructions and sport-specific stretches make them a great resource. Yoga classes are an excellent way to work on flexibility, but make sure to start with a beginner class.

7

Keeping Up in the Bedroom

The most distressing and potentially emasculating symptom of andropause is erection problems. The instantaneous boom in sales of the impotence drug Viagra®, which went from zero to well over a million in a couple of months, testifies to this fact. However, Viagra is so new that we aren't entirely sure of its side effects; and it is expensive, costing between $8 and $10 a pill.

Twenty percent of men complain of impotence by the time they are fifty-five, and that figure soars to more than 50 percent in seventy-five-year-olds. Because many men are reluctant to admit that they have a problem, they don't get the help they need to enjoy a satisfying sex life.

Great sex can make a man feel like a lusty teenager and it can play a role in turning back the aging clock. A healthy, loving relationship with your partner is enhanced by good sex. Studies show that whether we are loving and loved is a good predictor of how long we'll live.

In this chapter, you'll discover what causes those miraculous erections, and what can make them elusive as the years pass by. I'm also going to talk you through a wide array of solutions—from simple lifestyle changes to supplements to hormone replacement, as well as medical and surgical solutions—so that you can have a satisfying sex life at any age!

IT ISN'T ALL IN YOUR MIND

In the 1950s, the general consensus was that almost all erection problems were caused by anxiety. Although you may have read that the brain is the most important sex organ, some researchers believe that 85 percent of erection problems are due to the fact that something's physically awry. Before I tell you all the things that can go wrong, though, let's look at how it works when everything's running smoothly.

THE ANATOMY OF ERECTION AND EJACULATION

The penis is a rounded triangular cylinder within which are three spongelike chambers: two *corpora cavernosa* and one *corpus spongiosum.* Nerve fibers branch from the spinal cord at the lower back, or *sacrum,* and spread throughout the tissues of the male sex organs. In response to sexual stimulation, whether from actual sexual contact or the thought of it, these nerves send signals to the blood vessels of the penis. The arterioles (small arteries) that bring oxygenated blood into the penis open wider and the veins that take blood back to the rest of the body clamp down, so that more blood enters the penis than exits it. The corpora cavernosa and corpus spongiosum then become engorged with blood, the penis stiffens, and it's ready for action. This also happens three to five times, for twenty-five to thirty-five minutes each time, during a night's sleep in a healthy male. Nighttime erections can be thought of as a workout routine for the penis, keeping its tissues well oxygenated and nourished—the same thing we do for the body when we exercise.

With continued arousal or stimulation, erection becomes more intense, and contraction of muscles surrounding the base of the penis raises the internal pressure even higher. After ejaculation, the arterioles that have been opened wide constrict as the veins that have been constricted relax, so that excess blood is quickly pumped back into the general circulation and the penis becomes flaccid again.

Semen, the fluid expelled during ejaculation, is made up of sperm formed in the testicles and nutrient-rich, slightly basic (in pH) fluids from the seminal vesicles and prostate. When sexual arousal commences, sperm formed and stored in a tiny, tightly wound tubule within each testicle (the *epididymis*) pass into thick, muscular tubules (the *vas deferens*) that pump them up to the *seminal vesicles.* These vesicles and the *prostate gland* contribute fluids containing minerals, sugars, enzymes, prostaglandins (one of the body's chemical messengers), and immune factors. Sperm and seminal fluid continue along to the ejaculatory duct, where they wait for the powerful contractions that accompany orgasm to propel the approximately three milliliters of semen into the urethra and out of the penis. All this is part of the design that gets 300 million or so little packets of genetic material through their journey alive and well and able to fertilize the ovum.

Impotence is the inability to maintain an erection long enough to allow for satisfying intercourse. Diagnosis of impotence by a physician is made when a patient complains of consistent erectile failure for at least six months, or in more than half of his attempts to perform sexually. The causes of impotence fall into several categories, which I'll discuss in a moment.

Let's be careful to make the distinction between impotence and decreased *libido* (desire for sex). Impotence occurs when the man's anatomy doesn't operate correctly, although his libido may be strong. The loss of sexual desire may well be a physiological phenomenon caused by a drug's side effects or a hormone imbalance. Sexual desire that is repeatedly frustrated by an inability to perform can certainly lead to loss of libido.

If a man finds he is simply not as interested in sex as he'd like to be, it's a good indication that his androgen (male hormone) levels are low.

ARTERY DISEASE

The number one killer of American men—coronary artery disease—has effects throughout the body. If the vessels that feed the heart muscle are clogged, chances are very good that they are also clogged elsewhere in the body. Vessels in the brain that are affected by artery disease can close off blood flow and cause stroke. Vessels in the legs can also be affected, leading to a very painful condition called *peripheral vascular disease.* If arterioles into the penis are narrowed by cholesterol-filled plaques, the process of filling the spongy erectile tissues with blood takes considerably longer. Blood flow may not be adequate for full erection. Even if an erection is achieved under these conditions, it becomes less likely that it will remain hard for long. Studies show that high cholesterol and high insulin levels cause blood vessels to constrict, and getting these metabolic disorders under control through supplements, diet, and exercise can help restore potency in men whose erection problems can be traced back to narrowed blood vessels.

Even when the arteries function properly, the penile veins must also participate in the process that leads to erection. These veins may be "leaky" in men who smoke, are diabetics, or have arterial disease. In each of these cases, the blood leaks out of the penis back into the general circulation, thwarting attempts at intercourse.

DIABETES

Diabetics are at particularly high risk of impotence because of poor circulation. Fifty to 60 percent of diabetic males are impotent. Forty percent are unable to ejaculate normally, suffering from *retrograde ejaculation* (flow of semen into the bladder because the sphincter muscle that normally blocks sperm from entering the bladder doesn't close). Nerve damage is common in diabetics, and impotence can result if the neurotransmitters that cause erection aren't released in high enough concentrations. Clogged blood vessels are a common reason for erectile dysfunction in diabetics. Men with diabetes or severe artery disease often end up with hardening *(fibrosis)* of parts of the spongy erectile tissue, or wasting *(atrophy)* of the smooth muscle at the base of the penis that constricts during peak arousal.

PRESCRIPTION DRUGS

Many of the drugs prescribed to men with heart disease or diabetes are directly responsible for the ensuing impotence. According to Dr. Earl Mindell, author of *Prescription Alternatives,* impotence is a known side effect of many high blood pressure medications; antidepressants; antibiotics; antihistamines; weight-loss drugs such as fenfluramine; H2 blockers such as Tagamet and Zantac; heart drugs such as beta blockers, calcium channel blockers, ACE inhibitors, and angina drugs; painkillers, sedatives, tranquilizers, and sleeping pills; and prostate drugs. The SSRI antidepressants such as Prozac, Zoloft, and Effexor tend to maintain erections, but since they also tend to kill libido, they aren't much help. In fact, since they tend to create a false sense of emotional detachment, they tend to be "sex sinkers" for both men and women.

Impotence in men who use these drugs is usually due to the physiological side effects of the drug. For example, if blood pressure is artificially lowered by a drug, the amount of pressure required for the penis to become erect will be insufficient, and the erection may not occur.

Drugs That Can Cause Impotence

✔ Antidepressants, including monoamine oxidase inhibitors (MAOIs), Prozac and other selective serotonin reuptake inhibitors (SSRIs), and tricyclic antidepressants.

✔ Tranquilizers, sedatives, sleeping pills, narcotics, and hypnotics, including phenothiazines, benzodiazepines, meprobamate, and barbiturates.

✔ Estrogens and anti-androgens prescribed for prostate cancer or other problems; and drugs that can act as anti-androgens such as cimetidine (Tagamet), ketoconazole, and cyproterone acetate.

✔ Drugs used to treat enlarged prostate (BPH).

✔ Antihistamines used to treat colds and allergies.

✔ Heart drugs, including drugs that lower blood pressure, beta blockers, calcium channel blockers, ACE inhibitors, and angina drugs.

Source: *Prescription Alternatives* by Earl Mindell, R.Ph., Ph.D., and Virginia Hopkins. Reprinted with permission.

Recreational drugs can also have adverse effects on sexual performance. Marijuana causes a drop in testosterone levels; excessive alcohol consumption can lead to impotence due to increased levels of circulating estrogens; and smoking can cause arteries and veins to constrict, leak, or otherwise become diseased.

HORMONE IMBALANCE

Low levels of testosterone can contribute to impotence, but the research is inconclusive. The major effect of testosterone deficiency on sexuality seems to be loss of libido. Although testosterone replacement does help some impotent men regain what they've lost, there's no definitive proof that it works by enhancing erections. You know from chapter 3 that there are many other reasons to use testosterone replacement therapy, and your man might feel an improvement in libido and erections with therapy if his levels are low.

My guess is that in the near future, more attention will be paid to hormone *balance* in male impotence and infertility. Because of the abundant sources of xenoestrogen pollutants in our environment, men are carrying around a lot more estrogens than their bodies are designed to handle. This is already dramatically reflected in the animal world. Male mollusks, reptiles, amphibians, and birds are being born with dysfunctional reproductive systems. The water in and on which they live is contaminated by processed sewage that contains high levels of estrogen from the urine of women on birth control pills and hormone replacement therapy; by industrial waste; and by pesticides.

Humans are certainly being similarly affected by contaminated water and food. The powerful xenoestrogen DES (diethylstilbestrol), given to pregnant women to prevent miscarriage, was banned in humans once it was shown that the sons of these women had reduced testicular size and function. Eventually it was discovered that DES daughters have higher rates of cervical cancer, and DES sons have higher rates of testicular cancer. In spite of that, DES is still widely fed to livestock such as steers and hogs to fatten them up for market. Even the trace amounts found in the meat of such animals is enough to have an estrogenic, or feminizing, effect on males. This is why I so strongly encourage everyone to eat only hormone-free, pesticide-free, range-fed meat.

The prevalence of obesity also contributes to male hormonal imbalance, because estrogens are stored and manufactured in fat tissue in both sexes. If a man is carrying around extra fat, he has extra estrogen circulating in his body. The imbalance of estrogens with androgens (including testosterone and DHEA) literally makes him less male and decreases his potency.

PROSTATE SURGERY

If impotence began after surgery for prostate cancer or prostate enlargement—it's a common side effect—there is still an advantage in many of the therapies referred to in this chapter. Refer to chapter 8, "Protecting His Prostate," for a thorough discussion of this topic.

PSYCHOLOGICAL PROBLEMS

Most impotent men over fifty have both physical and psychological problems to cope with. Solutions begin when the person is able to speak openly and honestly to his doctor and his partner about his fears and feelings, and/or to seek counseling.

When the patient first sees a physician about impotence, the doctor will ask a lot of questions or have him fill out a questionnaire in order to determine the appropriate tests to administer. The form will include questions about whether he has nighttime erections, and what drugs he takes. A thorough physical exam will include a test of the reflex arc that causes erection, to rule out a neurological problem. This is an uncomfortable but brief procedure in which the doctor inserts one finger into the patient's anus and gently squeezes the tip of the penis. If the reflex arc is intact, the anal sphincter will contract.

Blood may be drawn to check levels of testosterone, prolactin, leutinizing hormone (LH), and follicle-stimulating hormone (FSH). The doctor may perform a Doppler study to make visible the blood vessels in the penis, or inject the penis with a smooth-muscle relaxant to see if an erection results; these tests are designed to discern whether impotence is a result of partly clogged blood vessels. The rate at which erection diminishes will also be considered, because a quickly waning erection is an indication that the veins leading out of the penis are leaky. The patient may be given instructions to perform a *nocturnal penile tumescence test* to evaluate whether his erection problems are physiological or psychological. (A simplified version can be done at home by snugly affixing a few stamps around the circumference of the penis while it's limp, and checking in the morning to see if the perforations between the stamps are torn.) Having plenty of good healthy erections during the night indicates nothing's the matter with the plumbing.

Once all the tests have been performed, the doctor will sit down and discuss treatment options.

SOLUTIONS TO THE PROBLEM OF IMPOTENCE

Treatments for impotence fall into several categories. There are non-medical, nonsurgical treatments that involve lifestyle change and nutritional or hormonal supplements. These solutions work best in milder cases that involve some level of blood vessel disease, which can be reversed with diet, exercise, and artery-opening supplements. Even without a diagnosis of atherosclerosis, impotence is a sign that circulation in the penis isn't as good as it could be. You can encourage the man in your life to do all he can to keep blood vessels clean of deposits. Refer to pages 174–175 for detailed information on how to deal naturally with blood vessel disease.

If decreased libido exists along with erection problems, the best approach is to have hormone levels tested and begin a course of natural hormone replacement therapy if it's needed. It is advisable for a man to wean himself off prescription drugs, if possible, with the help of a health professional. Here are some potent androgen-stimulating herbal remedies he can try as well.

- Yohimbine: a derivative of the bark of the yohimbine tree that has been patented for use as a prescription drug (Yocon,

Yohimbex). It's indicated for occasional use just before having sex. Its effectiveness has been proven beyond question by a decade of clinical research, and is safe as long as too much isn't taken at one time. It shouldn't be used more than once a week, because it has a potent stimulant effect throughout the body, and check first with your doctor if you have heart disease. Follow directions on the label.

- Ginkgo: dilates arteries to improve erectile function in those with mild blood vessel disease.

- Ginseng: a gentle overall stimulant that can lengthen duration and increase rigidity of erections. Ginseng and ginkgo can be used regularly: they both have a balancing and tonifying effect throughout the body.

- Wild oats *(Avena sativa)* and *Urtica dioica:* the anecdotal evidence from those who have tried these herbs for impotence is promising, but there's no significant clinical research yet to back up these claims.

- Damiana *(Turnera aphrodisiaca)* and saw palmetto: for a healthy prostate (see chapter 8).

- Ashwaghanda: an Indian tonic herb used traditionally to improve libido and sexual performance.

VACUUM CONSTRICTION DEVICES

These unpleasant-sounding plastic gizmos are one of the first-line therapies for impotence. A cylindrical chamber is placed over the penis and a vacuum is pulled to draw blood into erectile tissues. Once the penis is erect, a constriction band is placed around the base to maintain the erection throughout intercourse and orgasm. Men who have used this method enjoy its safety and effectiveness, but complain of awkwardness and lack of spontaneity. The tight rubber ring around the base of the penis can inhibit ejaculation in some men who use the vacuum device.

Vasoactive Drug Injection Therapy

"Ouch!" may be the initial response when anyone suggests injecting a drug into the penis to produce an erection. It's really not so bad, though; the needle is tiny, the same size used by diabetics for insulin injections. My patients say that once they are used to it, it is an easy and highly effective way to restore potency. These drugs work by stimulating production of *nitric oxide* (NO) within blood vessels. Nitric oxide has been generating a lot of interest in research circles lately because it quickly opens up blood vessels, allowing enhanced blood flow. The heart drug nitroglycerine, used to rapidly alleviate angina pains, works by the nitric oxide mechanism.

When these drugs (available only by prescription) are injected into the shaft of the penis, blood flow is increased; within ten to fifteen minutes, the penis is fully erect. The erection is then maintained for thirty to fifty minutes, even through orgasm.

Men with severe blood vessel disease, hemophilia, anemia, varicose veins in the penis, very poor eyesight, or coordination problems shouldn't use this method. An exact dose must be injected, and it should never be used more than once every two or three days. If the drug is overused or too high a dose is injected, a painful, persistent erection *(priapism)* can occur, which, in the worst-case scenario, may permanently damage the penis. In any case, it may create a strong aversion to using it again. It may take a few tries to find the perfect dose, but he should always start with low doses.

If the doctor prescribes prostaglandin-E, phentolamine, phenoxybenzamine, or papaverine (Caverject), he may also prescribe a medication to take in case of accidental overdose. Side effects of penile injection may include bruising or infection at the injection site, temporary dizziness or sudden drop in blood pressure, or ejaculatory difficulties.

Also available are intraurethral (a small pellet inserted into the tip of the penis) and topical (rubbed onto the penis) versions of these vasoactive agents.

An Erection Aid You Can Take in the Form of a Pill

The drug Viagra (sildenafil) has become the impotence drug of choice all over the world; it has also become the subject of numerous tasteless jokes about erectile dysfunction. Unlike other erection aids, Viagra doesn't automatically bring about erection when it's used. Taken an hour before intercourse, it potentiates the erectile response to erotic stimulation by relaxing the smooth-muscle cells that line the penile arteries. Side effects may include diarrhea and headache. It's most effective in partially impotent men. There have been dozens of deaths associated with the use of Viagra, but it's difficult to say whether the deaths were caused by the drug itself or by the stress of newly rediscovered sex on an old heart.

Penile Prosthesis and Other Surgical Approaches

The therapy of last resort is the penile prosthesis. Some prostheses are semirigid or hinged, so that they are always erect and can be folded up when you're going about your day; others are inflatable. Modern medical technology has made penile prostheses very comfortable and user-friendly. The surgeon implants the prosthesis through a small incision in the scrotum. Some implants include a fluid-filled chamber implanted into the abdomen or scrotum, and the fluid is pumped into the prosthesis before intercourse. A valve holds the fluid in the implant until after intercourse, at which time the fluid is released through the valve back into the chamber. Because implantation is a surgical procedure, there are many potential complications, including scarring and infection. Still, severely impotent men who have penile implants are generally very pleased with them, because they work consistently.

Surgeons are now experimenting with the same sort of bypass surgeries used to get oxygenated blood around blockages in the arteries to the heart muscle. Penile bypass surgeries are still in the experimental stages, and if they become an accepted therapy for impotence they will probably serve as one of the "last resort" solutions, once all other, less invasive options have been tried.

OTHER KINDS OF MALE REPRODUCTIVE DYSFUNCTION

Some men have adequate erections but complain of premature ejaculation (uncontrolled ejaculation before or soon after penetration), delayed ejaculation, or retrograde ejaculation (where semen flows backward into the bladder).

Premature ejaculation is best handled with counseling and sexual techniques designed to blunt the man's responsiveness. Thick condoms can dull sensation just enough to delay ejaculation. The *squeeze technique* is a desensitization technique: when he feels ejaculation approaching, you squeeze the head of his penis, with the thumb underneath and the index and second fingers along the curve at the top where the head meets the shaft. The erection will probably go down a bit as well. When it feels as if it's under control, resume your activities, and repeat the cycle several times.

Retrograde ejaculation, where the bladder sphincter has lost some tone and semen goes into the bladder, is a bit harder to fix. It doesn't interfere with the sensations of ejaculation, however, and some fluid (semen) is released out of the body during ejaculation. This problem is indicated by a low volume of ejaculate and urine that tends to be cloudy after sex. Unless you're trying to conceive a child, though, it shouldn't stand in the way of a satisfying sex life.

INFERTILITY

Fifteen to 20 percent of American couples are unable to accomplish what so many teenagers and young adults take great pains to avoid—making a baby. Infertility is becoming an issue for many middle-aged men in second marriages with younger women, or those who are trying to conceive later in life. The number of couples seeking therapy for infertility is rising rapidly.

A diagnosis of infertility is made if a couple is having frequent, unprotected sex yet cannot conceive within one year. Male infertility can be caused by a number of factors, including:

- low sperm counts
- problems with sperm motility
- decreased volume or increased viscosity of semen
- scarring from infections of the genitourinary tract
- low androgen levels, resulting in testicular atrophy and impaired sperm production
- prostate disease
- antibodies to their own sperm (generally due to obstructed passage of sperm out of the body)
- varicocele (varicose vein in the penis)

Women may be infertile from delaying childbearing; blocked fallopian tubes, which prevent the egg from reaching the uterus; endometriosis; or hormone imbalances. Women in the last decade of reproductive life have more early miscarriages (spontaneous abortions) and have many menstrual cycles that don't include ovulation (anovulatory cycles).

The breakdown of causes of infertility, with consideration of what could go wrong with either sex, is as follows:

- 15 to 20 percent from ovulatory dysfunction (eggs not being released from the ovaries)

- 30 to 40 percent from scarring and adhesions in the fallopian tubes due to endometriosis, pelvic inflammatory disease (PID), or other infections of the female reproductive tract
- 30 to 40 percent due to male factors listed above
- 5 to 10 percent due to disorders of the mucus of the cervix or semen, or to the man having antibodies to his own sperm

In 10 to 15 percent of cases, no cause can be found. Twenty to 40 percent of couples have more than one of these causes.

A FEW THINGS TO TRY BEFORE SEEING A DOCTOR

If conception isn't happening, and the problem isn't erectile dysfunction, there are a few things you can try to improve your chances. Medical fertility evaluations and treatments are time-consuming, stressful, expensive (usually not covered by medical insurance), and don't always work, especially for older couples. That's why it's a good idea to try these tactics before resorting to medical interventions.

First, think about making some lifestyle changes. Smoking and liberal consumption of alcohol are "no-nos" for couples who are trying to conceive. Frequent use of marijuana will also interfere with conception. If the marijuana is tainted with pesticides, as it often is, the health of the fetus is negatively affected. Consume a healthy, additive-free diet, with organic veggies and free-range meats, eggs, and dairy. Some couples find that giving up dairy products altogether makes a difference. Try to phase out medications and limit exposure to toxins. Stress reduction is important for both partners. The woman's body is wise: it will not conceive if it perceives her environment to be too dangerous for her to carry a child to term.

The man can avoid wearing snug, brief-style underwear and forgo frequent hot baths. Raised temperatures lower sperm counts. Think of how the testicles respond to a swim in cold water—they contract into the body, right? That's how they conserve heat. Normal testicles, when a man is comfortably warm, hang a little lower. Keeping the testicles against his body with snug underwear or pants keeps their temperature artificially high and deactivates sperm. (Some boys are born with undescended testicles, and if this isn't surgically remedied before the age of six, the seminiferous tubules are destroyed by the high temperatures within the body cavity.) Ditto for the hot tub or sauna. He can try boxer shorts or boxer briefs (a jockey short–boxer hybrid); stay away from Spandex shorts and skintight jeans.

Too-frequent intercourse and/or masturbation can result in depletion of sperm reserves. You and your partner can determine the day of each month when your ovulation takes place. Conserve his sperm for a few days at a time during your fertile period by refraining from intercourse. Then, have intercourse every forty-eight hours during this time. Obviously, intercourse that's too infrequent doesn't bode well for conception, either.

Some medical treatments damage the male reproductive system. Unfortunately, there's not much you can do to reverse this damage, but at least you'll know what might happen to his fertility and you can plan accordingly. Chemotherapy for lymphomas, leukemia, sarcomas, or testicular cancer can destroy the cells that manufacture sperm and his sperm counts may never regain their pretreatment levels. If he has ever had mumps affecting the testicles *(mumps orchitis),* venereal diseases like gonorrhea or syphilis, or some other infection affecting the epididymis, there may have been permanent damage. Surgery in or around the genitourinary tract can result in infertility, ejaculation problems, or impotence. Prescription drugs that decrease the body's natural androgen levels and anabolic steroids used by weightlifters can suppress sperm production.

Low levels of androgens can be a contributing factor in infertility. You already know how much androgen replacement can do for his health; improving fertility is a bonus if that's what you're after.

MEDICAL EVALUATION OF INFERTILITY

If you and your partner are having problems conceiving after a year of trying, each of you should undergo a complete physical exam. A complete history will be taken, including a sexual history. Don't be embarrassed—answer in as much detail as possible and remember, the doctor has heard it all before! Diagnostic tests should include analysis of semen in the man and vaginal mucosa in the woman, and evaluation of both partners' reproductive organs.

EVERYTHING YOU ALWAYS WANTED TO KNOW ABOUT SEMEN ANALYSIS

Your physician will obtain two or three samples of ejaculate over a one- to two-month period. You'll be instructed to abstain from sex for a couple of days beforehand. Masturbation into a sterile container at the doctor's office is one option, or you can have intercourse at home using a special silicone condom and bring the sample in within an hour. The lab assesses the sperm's swimming ability and the viscosity (thickness) of the semen. The necessary components of semen are all accounted for.

The sperm cells themselves are examined for abnormalities, and sperm count is determined. Average sperm count in a fertile male is between 60 and 80 million per milliliter of ejaculate, but the likelihood of conception doesn't diminish until the count goes below 20 million per milliliter. If the sperm are excellent swimmers and have all the necessary ingredients for penetration of the egg, sperm counts as low as 5 or 10 million per milliliter can hit the mark. Semen viscosity can also affect fertility; if there's too little or too much fluid, sperm can't get where they need to go. In some men, sperm clump up or orient themselves in patterns that prevent efficient swimming.

Infection, intense physical exercise, or illness can kill off sperm. If sperm are abnormal or sperm count is low, and this isn't attributable to any contact with chemicals or drugs harmful to the male reproductive system, a thorough evaluation of hormone levels is the next step. A test that evaluates the ability of sperm to survive the journey through the woman's reproductive system, called a postcoital test, can be done in the middle of her monthly cycle.

If sperm counts are low or there are no sperm in the ejaculate, but hormone levels and testicular function are adequate, the problem is probably varicocele, retrograde ejaculation, or some blockage in the ductwork. Microsurgery or other high-tech interventions can have great results in these instances. You can opt for in vitro fertilization if the man doesn't want to have surgery or if surgery won't solve the problems.

In the case of retrograde ejaculation, sperm usually have to be harvested to fertilize the ovum in a petri dish. Baking soda is taken by mouth so that the urine is less acidic and doesn't immediately kill sperm.

As I've said, the process of infertility evaluation is intensive and expensive. Find a doctor you trust and ask plenty of questions, be supportive of your partner, and seek counseling if the stress threatens to get the best of either of you.

8

Protecting His Prostate

The prostate, a walnut-sized gland that wraps around the urethra just below the bladder, can cause a lot of trouble during the second half of a man's life. The more a man learns about all that can go awry in this small organ, the more he's likely to feel as though he's got a ticking time bomb lodged in his genitourinary tract. The prostate swells and closes in on the urethra in multitudes of men over fifty. This affliction, *benign prostatic hyperplasia,* or BPH, plagues 50 percent of fifty-year-old men, 70 percent of seventy-year-old men, and 80 percent of eighty-year-old men. Prostate cancer is the most common male cancer and the second most common cause of cancer-related death in men.

The good news is that a lot can be done to maintain the health of the prostate throughout the forties, fifties, sixties, and beyond. With the appropriate diet, supplements, and exercise, BPH can be prevented, treated, or reversed. The risk of prostate cancer is also linked to lifestyle choices, in ways that are not as well understood.

SOME PROSTATE GLAND ANATOMY AND PHYSIOLOGY

The *urethra* is a tube with eliminatory and reproductive functions. (See Figure 8.1.) It carries urine from the kidneys, where it's made, down to the bladder, within which it's held by a sphincter muscle. When it's time to urinate, the sphincter releases and urine drains out of the bladder through the urethra, which carries it out through the penis. Smooth muscle around the bladder allows a man to control urine flow and push out those last few drops. Semen also passes through this tube during ejaculation, propelled by muscle contractions from the vas deferens, and this is where the prostate kicks in.

The prostate gland makes a nutrient-rich, bicarbonate-rich fluid that nourishes and protects sperm. When orgasm occurs, the well-muscled prostate pumps its contribution into the urethra, where it mingles with sperm from the testes and the fluid from the seminal vesicles (also rich in vitamins and sugars).

The secretions of the vagina are slightly acidic, and would kill off sperm immediately if the prostate did not contribute bicarbonate to buffer the acid. Zinc, proteins, and sugars give sperm enough resources to survive for up to three days in the female reproductive tract, just waiting to connect with that elusive ovum.

THE AGING PROSTATE

The growth of the prostate gland is regulated by several hormones, the most important of these being the androgens, or male hormones. When rats are castrated, their prostates shrink; when androgens are replaced, the prostate grows back to its original size. Other hormones, including insulin, IGF-1, the estrogens, luteinizing hormone, and prolactin, also have roles in the maintenance of a healthy prostate.

Figure 8.1 The Male Reproductive System.

Side View

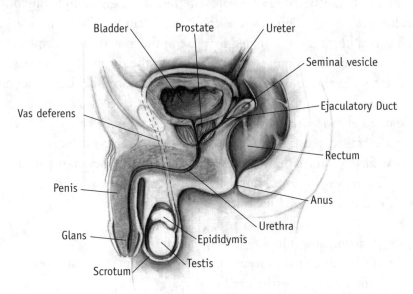

Front View

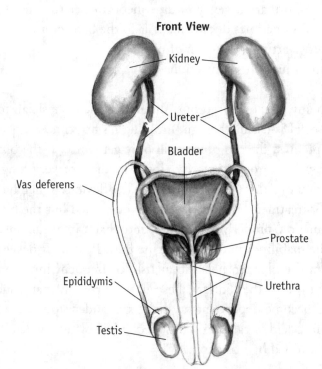

When the balance of these hormones changes during andropause, the result can be BPH. The prostate begins to grow, and sometimes closes in on the urethra, squeezing it partly closed. This appears to be due to a hormone-stimulated increase in the growth or multiplication of prostate cells, along with a decrease in the death of prostate cells. Changes in the conversion of one form of a hormone to another and changes in the number of prostate hormone receptors cause the prostate to expand. BPH and prostate cancer can both be traced back to uncontrolled prostate cell growth. It's comparable to the parking lot that fills up, but more cars keep coming in, and they start parking illegally, narrowing and eventually blocking the flow of traffic.

Symptoms of BPH include:

- Starting and stopping during urination
- Frequent urination (especially if sleep is interrupted several times a night by the need to urinate)
- Feelings of urinary urgency or urge incontinence (one has to go badly and sometimes doesn't make it to the bathroom)
- Difficulty starting the stream of urine
- Frequent urinary tract infections

Men with any of these symptoms should see their physician for an evaluation. BPH is usually benign, meaning it's not cancerous, but if it is left to progress the symptoms will only get worse. If the bladder has to force urine through a partly closed urethra for very long, the muscle surrounding this organ can become less flexible. When he does finally go for treatment, the blockage may be cleared but the bladder may not function properly anymore—and that can mean incontinence, or the inability to hold back urine flow. If urine is never fully drained from the bladder, he's also at risk for frequent infections. If urine backs up into the kidneys, he can end up with major kidney damage and become dependent on dialysis. Bladder stones, made of crystallized uric acid or calcium, can collect in the bladder when it isn't completely emptied by urination.

WHAT TO EXPECT AT THE DOCTOR'S OFFICE

Every man's favorite procedure, the digital rectal exam, and a *prostate-specific antigen* (PSA) test are indicated when a man arrives with complaints of any of the above symptoms. (The PSA test is used mainly to look for prostate cancer, and I'll discuss that in more detail later on.) If the physician deduces from symptoms or during the rectal exam that the prostate is closing off the flow of urine, a referral to a urologist is next. During the week or so before the appointment with the urologist, the patient needs to jot down his symptoms as he experiences them; this will help the doctor decide upon the best treatment options.

At the appointment with the urologist, the patient will be asked about symptoms. Honest answers are crucial: any shyness can endanger his health in the long run. There will be tests to check for blood or infection in the urine, and tests of strength and reflexes to rule out nerve damage from other causes such as diabetes, multiple sclerosis, spinal stenosis (impingement of tissues on the nerves that run to the urinary tract), or Parkinson's disease. There are a few tests that involve the insertion of catheters into the penis; a local anesthetic is administered first. Ultrasound and X-rays are sometimes used in a prostate evaluation.

SURGICAL TREATMENT OPTIONS FOR BPH

The best initial response to BPH is watchful waiting, during which time symptoms are carefully monitored. If this is what the doctor advises, the patient will also be told to avoid over-the-counter decongestants because they cause the muscles in the prostate and bladder to tense up. He'll also be advised to avoid drinking lots of fluids before bed. When he goes in for checkups, he'll be evaluated again to determine how the prostate enlargement is progressing.

If the prostate has enlarged to the point where it seriously interferes with the ability to urinate, the "gold standard" of treatments is TURP—*transurethral resection of the prostate.* A catheter is introduced into the prostate through the urethra. The tissue at the center of the gland is pulled away and removed, and the rest of the gland is left intact. The removed tissue is biopsied for cancerous cells. TURP is done under spinal or epidural anesthetic—drugs are given intravenously or by injection into the spine to numb the lower half of the body. More than half of men who have had TURP report "dry" ejaculation when they resume sexual activity, but this doesn't appear to adversely affect performance or change the way orgasm feels.

If the prostate is very enlarged, or if there are other medical contraindications to the use of the catheter, the surgeon will probably perform an *open prostatectomy* in which the swollen tissues are removed through an incision in the belly. A vasectomy is usually performed along with the open prostatectomy to prevent inflammation of the epididymis (tubes that carry sperm toward the urethra). Common side effects of this surgery are retrograde ejaculation—sperm are ejaculated into the bladder rather than out of the penis—and impotence.

Unfortunately, these surgeries are not permanent solutions. Only the prostate cells that directly interfere with urinary flow are removed. Remaining prostate tissue continues to expand, and the procedure generally has to be repeated. The insertion of an *intraurethral stent,* a stiff, small section of plastic "pipe" that keeps the urethra open even if the prostate presses in on it, may help preserve the openness of the urinary tract after surgery, although it can trigger scar tissue formation that causes the same problems.

There are several other medical treatments for BPH. Heat, laser, ultrasound, and microwaves appear effective in burning away the swollen parts of the prostate; they selectively kill cells, which are then sloughed off and absorbed by the body. All of these approaches have side effects, and none are permanent solutions.

DRUGS FOR PROSTATE ENLARGEMENT

The widely accepted theory of what causes BPH involves the conversion of testosterone to *dihydrotestosterone* (DHT) by the enzyme *5-alpha-reductase*. DHT is responsible for carrying out many of the duties of testosterone throughout the body, and is ten times more active in the prostate than is testosterone. In the male fetus, DHT is needed for the development of the male reproductive system. Hermaphroditism, a birth defect in which the genitalia are ambiguous—part male, part female—can be the result when there is a deficiency of 5-alpha-reductase. DHT plays an important role in the development and upkeep of the properly functioning prostate gland. By latching onto specialized receptors, DHT stimulates the creation of a particular genetic code that pieces together the proteins that make up the prostate cells. In men with congenital or inborn 5-alpha-reductase deficiency, the prostate remains very small throughout life. These men also tend to have sparse body hair and don't lose the hair on their heads.

Conventional medicine sees DHT as the source of prostate problems, a major cause of both BPH and prostate cancer. Drugs that block the action of 5-alpha-reductase do have the effect of shrinking the prostate by 20 to 30 percent. Finasteride (Proscar), a 5-alpha-reductase inhibitor, has become conventional medicine's drug of choice for mild cases of BPH. Unfortunately, it only works in about one-third of those who take it, but when it does it can slow the progression of BPH for at least three years. A minority of men experience impotence as a side effect, but potency returns when the drug is discontinued. One positive side effect some men experience with finasteride treatment is the slowing or halting of hair loss. (See chapter 9, "Keeping His Hair on His Head," for more on this topic.)

There are many other hormones involved in prostate gland maintenance, however, and researchers are examining several of them to try to better define the causes of and cures for BPH. Prolactin, the hormone that causes a pregnant woman's breasts to start making milk, and which is made in small amounts in men, has potent growth effects on the prostate. Prolactin levels tend to rise with age and may contribute to BPH.

Luteinizing hormone–releasing hormone (LHRH) comes from the hypothalamus in the brain and stimulates the release of luteinizing hormone (LH) from the pituitary. LH acts on testes in men and ovaries in women, stimulating the formation of androgens and estrogens. Excessive LHRH has been shown to cause excessive growth of prostate tissue, and studies are being performed to see whether LHRH-blocking drugs might be a good option for some cases of BPH. LHRH *agonists*—drugs that enhance LHRH secretion—seem to cause a paradoxical decrease in this hormone, and drugs that have this effect are also being studied.

THE EFFECTS OF ESTROGEN AND PROGESTERONE ON THE PROSTATE

Of particular interest in current prostate research is the role of estrogens. These female hormones have powerful opposing or reducing effects on androgen levels in men, as well as a direct effect on the prostate gland. One of the primary roles of estrogen in the body is to stimulate cell growth, which is exactly what we don't want happening in excess in the prostate gland. Sex hormone–binding globulin (SHBG) appears to have an important role in this interaction. I'm predicting that this research will lead to some significant breakthroughs in our understanding of prostate enlargement and prostate cancer.

Thanks to pervasive pollution, most American men have been exposed to powerful environmental estrogens, known as xenoestrogens, since before birth (see chapter 3 for details), and their prostates have extra receptors for estrogen because of this excessive exposure.

Overweight men convert more of the testosterone in their bodies into estrogens (a process referred to in scientific circles as *peripheral aromatization*), and as a result their estrogen loads rise. When a man's hormonal balances begin to go through other changes during andropause, his prostate is especially sensitive to the cooperative growth-promoting effects of estrogens, SHBG, and DHT.

Progesterone is a hormone made in the most copious amounts by the placenta when a woman is pregnant. Women also make progesterone when they ovulate during their menstrual cycles, and both sexes make some in their adrenal glands. Progesterone is not a sex hormone, meaning that it does not confer male or female attributes. In men and women it is a biochemical precursor to nearly all the steroid hormones, including the cortisones, DHEA, androstenedione, the estrogens, and testosterone. Progesterone also has the direct effect of reducing or moderating the growth-promoting effects of estrogen, and it may reduce the growth-promoting effects of DHT. Progesterone also keeps prolactin levels in check, and lowers levels of LH.

I have found progesterone to be very useful for treating prostate enlargement, and I have spoken to many other doctors who agree. I have also heard reports of the use of natural progesterone cream to reverse prostate cancer.

The best way to use progesterone is as a cream. It is easy to find in health-food stores. I recommend obtaining a cream that contains at least 450 milligrams of progesterone (*not* diosgenin, *Dioscorea,* or wild yam extract) per ounce of cream. A man can apply about one-eighth of a teaspoon directly to the scrotum and perineum area (between the scrotum and anus) daily. Find a cream that includes only progesterone and vitamin E as its active ingredients.

I strongly discourage the use of oral progesterone. If a man applies progesterone cream on the skin in small amounts, he gets a local response, which is what is needed. As soon as a man takes oral progesterone in capsule form, his digestive system and liver get involved, and we don't know the effects of that on men.

You should know that the use of progesterone to treat BPH and prostate cancer is not approved by the FDA, nor by anyone of mainstream status in scientific or medical circles, for that matter. At this time, its benefits are strictly anecdotal (by word of mouth), theoretical, and experimental. As a medical doctor I cannot recommend its use, but I can tell you that if I personally had prostate enlargement, I would try saw palmetto first, and if that didn't work I'd try the progesterone. If I had prostate cancer, the first thing I would try would be progesterone.

If you'd like a detailed description of progesterone and how it functions in women, find the best-selling book *What Your Doctor May Not Tell You About Menopause,* by John R. Lee, M.D., and then show the man in your life the chapters relevant to him.

USING DRUGS FOR THE PROSTATE

Drugs that relax the smooth muscle that surrounds the urethra and prostate may relieve urinary symptoms of BPH. These drugs, called *alpha-adrenergic blockers,* include prazosin (Minipress), tamsulosin (Flomax), terazosin (Hytrin), and doxasozin (Cardura). They are also used to treat high blood pressure. Some of the side effects of these alpha-adrenergic blockers include dizziness, very low blood pressure, and fast heartbeat (tachycardia), and they are hard on the liver.

PROTECTING THE PROSTATE WITHOUT DRUGS AND SURGERY

We've come a long way from the standard nineteenth-century therapy for prostate enlargement—castration—and there are some reliable natural alternatives to medical therapy when it comes to protecting the prostate. I've mentioned the use of natural progesterone. In Germany and Austria, physicians use plant medicines as the first treatment of choice in 90 percent of cases of mild to moderate BPH.

A whole-foods diet based on organic vegetables, fruits, and whole grains is the most important building block of a prostate-healing regimen. It is also important to keep a man's intake of environmental estrogens to a minimum and balance his hormone levels so the herbal remedies can do their gentle healing work. It may also help him to decrease or eliminate his alcohol consumption.

SAW PALMETTO AND OTHER NATURAL BPH REMEDIES

Saw Palmetto
The berries of the saw palmetto plant (*Serenoa repens,* or dwarf palm plant) have been used for decades in the treatment of BPH. In one study of 1,098 patients, saw palmetto extract and the prescription 5-alpha-reductase inhibitor finasteride (Proscar) had equally beneficial effects on BPH symptoms, with saw palmetto patients reporting far fewer adverse effects on libido and potency. Saw palmetto also has much less of a side effect on the wallet, being a third or less of the price of finasteride. Dozens of other studies corroborate this. Saw palmetto extract is a natural DHT antagonist, preventing its formation and its binding to the prostate, and may also inhibit the conversion of testosterone to estrogen. It's rich in essential fats that support the health of the prostate. The dose is 160 to 320 milligrams of saw palmetto berry extract twice per day as a capsule or liquid. There are many good natural formulas available for the prostate that include saw palmetto and other nutrients discussed in this chapter.

Beta-Sitosterol
Beta-sitosterol, a mixture of plant steroid extracts (phytosterols) derived from the saw palmetto berry, has shown great therapeutic

promise. In one study published in the British medical journal *Lancet,* 200 patients were either treated with 60 milligrams per day of beta-sitosterol (Harzol) or given a placebo. Those who took Harzol for six months had significant improvement in symptoms of BPH. As with most botanical medicines, clinical testing hasn't been rigorous enough to allow its acceptance into the conventional medical/pharmaceutical arsenal against prostate enlargement, but that shouldn't stop a man from trying it!

Nettle Root and Pygeum

Herbs called nettle root and *Pygeum africanum* are often included in saw palmetto formulas. *Pygeum africanum,* derived from the African plum plant, is another well-known botanical remedy for BPH. He can try a dose of 30 to 75 milligrams per day. Nettle root *(urtica dioica)* functions as an anti-inflammatory that seems to be specific to the prostate gland at a dosage of about 120 milligrams twice a day. (The amounts contained in formulas may vary from these recommended doses. Experiment and find the formula that works best.)

Ginseng

Animal studies of *Panax ginseng* yielded results of reduced prostate size and increased testosterone levels in subjects. This is a good indication that ginseng blocks the growth-promoting actions of DHT (by blocking conversion from testosterone) and estrogens. He should take enough of the capsules or tincture forms of ginseng to get 25 to 50 milligrams of ginsenosides per day, information that should be found on the product's label.

Zinc

There are high concentrations of zinc in prostate tissues. For BPH, supplement with 30 milligrams per day of zinc for up to six months, and after that make sure he's getting at least 10 to 15 milligrams per day.

OTHER HEALTHY PROSTATE SUPPLEMENTS

Some men find that taking a vitamin B₆ supplement helps reduce prostate enlargement. Since this vitamin is inextricably involved in the conversion of hormones, it's important for hormone balance. Start out with 100 milligrams per day for a month, and then maintain on 50 milligrams daily.

Pumpkin seeds are also found in many prostate formula supplements. They contain zinc and important essential fatty acids, which are important in reducing inflammation. If he enjoys the taste of pumpkin seeds, he can munch on a handful a few times a week.

HYDROTHERAPY

For symptom relief when the prostate is causing urinary problems, a hot sitz bath is helpful. Fill the tub or a sitz bath (a container that you sit in) with hot water, just enough to cover the genital area, and sit for three to ten minutes. This should soothe inflamed, constricted prostate and urethral smooth muscle. Following the hot sitz bath, sponge the genital and perineal area with cool water. (He shouldn't do this if you're trying to become pregnant, because heat kills sperm.)

PROSTATE CANCER

Twenty percent of all newly diagnosed cancers in the United States are cancers of the prostate gland; it's the most common cancer affecting American men. One in ten men can expect to develop prostate cancer in his lifetime. Fortunately, it is one of the slowest-growing cancers, and since it tends to show up primarily in old age, most men die from something else before the prostate cancer kills them.

The symptoms of early prostate cancer are similar to those seen in BPH: urinary hesitancy, frequent urination, interruption of urine flow, and so on. That's why it's important to have these symptoms checked as soon as they are noticed. There may also be back, hip, pelvis, or thigh pain; impotence; blood in the urine or semen; or a decrease in the volume of fluid expelled during ejaculation. Once symptoms like these are present, it's likely that the cancer has grown to a size that will require aggressive treatment.

THE PSA TEST

One way to detect prostate cancer is with a *PSA* test. PSA (prostate-specific antigen) is an enzyme manufactured in the prostate, and levels of this enzyme tend to be elevated in the blood of men with prostate problems. It has become a screening test that is now administered routinely to men over 40, and it's part of the reason that prostate cancer is becoming more prevalent—it's detected more often and earlier in its progression.

The downside of PSA testing is that it has a very high false-positive rate, meaning that as much as 70 percent of the time the test may come back positive when in reality it is normal. Personally, I would not consider having any type of prostate cancer treatment until I had had at least three positive tests with at least two different labs. PSA tests also have a high false-negative rate, meaning they don't show cancer even when it is present.

A normal PSA test result will show less than 4 nanograms of prostate-specific antigen per milliliter of blood serum (nanograms per milliliter). A very general interpretation of a PSA test higher than 4 nanograms per milliliter would be as follows: Every increase of 0.3 nanograms per milliliter above that level indicates one gram of hyperplastic tissue (excessive growth) in the prostate, while every increase of 3 nanograms per milliliter above that level indicates one gram of cancerous tissue in the prostate. There are many other considerations in reading a PSA test, but in general, the higher the PSA level, the more likely the man has prostate cancer. Slight elevations generally indicate BPH.

Because PSA is specific to prostate but not necessarily for cancer, a PSA levels can be high for reasons besides the presence of cancer. To make things even more confusing, about one-quarter of men who have prostate cancer have *low* PSA levels. In men with PSA levels between 4 and 10, about 25 percent have cancer. About 65 percent of men with PSA levels over 10 turn out to have cancer. All this is to say, never depend on PSA readings alone to make a diagnosis of cancer.

Statistics show that older men with high PSA levels who opt for prostate surgery have a higher death rate than older men who do nothing. Since prostate cancer is such a slow-growing cancer, "watchful waiting" is now the standard of care recommended by most physicians. Impotence and incontinence are common side effects of prostate surgery, so it's not something to take lightly.

On the other hand, the judicious use of prostate screening means that physicians are seeing fewer men with previously undetected, advanced prostate cancer. Since 1986, the incidence of widely metastasized (spread throughout the body) prostate cancer has decreased by more than 60 percent.

If the test comes out positive, proceed with extreme caution and be conservative. Once a man is rendered impotent or incontinent by surgery there's no going back.

What If My PSA Test Comes Back Positive?

An elevation of PSA is not a sure sign of prostate cancer. It could also mean BPH or prostatitis (an infection of the prostate). Some men with perfectly healthy prostates have elevated PSAs. A transrectal ultrasound and needle biopsy, along with the digital rectal exam, will help the urologist determine what's wrong and what the best treatments might be.

Prostate cancer is detectable at a much earlier stage than ever before—long before the doctor can feel cancerous lumps during a digital rectal exam. Men with very early prostate cancer who are being diagnosed and treated aggressively with removal of the gland (radical prostatectomy) may well be better off with watchful waiting. Some prostate cancers grow so slowly that they never pose any risk of spreading, while others grow rapidly.

THE AMAS TEST

Another option a man has if he has high PSA levels is to have an AMAS (antimalignan antibody in serum), which is an FDA-approved, patented, and generic test for even the smallest malignant cancer of any kind, anywhere in the body. The test has an accuracy rate of 95 percent, and 99 percent on the second test, which is much more reliable than a PSA test.

The AMAS test involves a substance called malignan, which is released by cancer cells and is recognized by the immune system, which responds with antibodies. Anytime malignan is released, the immune system responds with antibodies called antimalignans, which are detected by the AMAS test.

After receiving a high PSA reading, it's well worth it to get an AMAS test to rule out a malignancy and avoid a biopsy or other invasive surgery. If there are symptoms of prostate enlargement, it's probably a good idea to get an AMAS test every year. To order an AMAS test kit, call Oncolab at 1-800-922-8378 and leave your name, address and phone number.

HORMONAL THERAPY FOR PROSTATE CANCER

Hormonal therapy, also referred to as "androgen ablation" and "chemical castration," is employed when cancer can't be eliminated by surgery, radiation, or cryoablation (freezing). Prostate cancer cells are

stimulated to grow and spread by androgens, so it follows that blocking androgen action slows their growth. Proscar, also used for BPH,
blocks conversion of testosterone to DHT, while a drug called cyproterone acetate blocks the release of LHRH (the hypothalamic hormone that stimulates the formation of testosterone in the testicles).
Hydroxyflutamide, casodex, and nilutamide block androgen action at
the cellular level. Synthetic estrogens are sometimes used to counteract androgens in advanced prostate cancer, but to my mind this is
putting the fox in charge of the henhouse, since estrogens also stimulate cell growth and are known promoters of reproductive cancers in
women. Removal of the testicles (*orchidectomy* or *castration*) significantly but only temporarily slows the growth of metastatic prostate
cancer.

With any treatment that brings androgen levels way down, there are
multiple side effects: impotence, loss of libido, and growth of breast
tissue (gynecomastia). Once these treatments are necessary, however,
it may be more a matter of prolonging survival and relieving pain than
preserving potency. Another caveat of androgen ablation is that prostate cancers can mutate and develop the ability to grow and spread
without the aid of androgens.

As I mentioned in the section on BPH, I have heard a number of
reports from other physicians that the use of progesterone cream on
patients' scrotums and perineums successfully reversed high PSA test
results. As I said, if I were diagnosed with prostate cancer, I would certainly give progesterone cream a try before surgery or drugs. You can
reread the section on BPH for the details of progesterone use.

It's also extremely important to minimize exposure to environmental estrogens, a topic that was covered on pages 41–42. Cancer is a
complex entity with thousands of manifestations, all of which share
two important characteristics: They multiply and spread unfettered by
the normal regulatory mechanisms that keep cell growth in check, and
they are *undifferentiated,* meaning that they don't perform any of the
specific functions of a body's cells. That's why cancer kills: Healthy

cells that perform vital functions are replaced by cancer cells, which are good for nothing but multiplying and spreading, utilizing the energy and space needed by healthy cells. That is why it is so important to avoid estrogen, which encourages undifferentiated cell growth, and why progesterone, which encourages cells to grow *toward* differentiation and opposes the growth-promoting actions of estrogen, is going to help.

PREVENTING PROSTATE CANCER

Most cancers are directly related to lifestyle and dietary factors, and prostate cancer is no exception. In studies of different world populations, the incidence of prostate cancer is highest in those with a "Western" diet and way of life—processed foods, sugar, rancid fats, few fresh fruits and vegetables, high levels of stress, and very little exercise. When men from Asia and South America, where risk is statistically low, migrate to the United States and adapt to our Western lifestyle, their statistical risk becomes identical to ours within a few generations.

Cancer cells can lie dormant for years, perhaps never growing enough to become clinically significant. If something triggers them— for example, a poor lifestyle or shifting hormone levels during andropause—they can get out of control. An interesting point specific to prostate cancer is that the incidence of early, nonaggressive, localized cancer of the prostate is about the same all over the world, but in Westernized countries it's more likely to grow to dangerous dimensions.

Most studies on possible dietary links show a strong relationship between fats and prostate cancer. The highest incidence of prostate cancer in the United States is in areas where consumption of meat and dairy products are high. There is some controversy about which fats increase risk, but I would suggest that you take special care to avoid the trans-fatty-acids, also called hydrogenated oils, which are synthetic fats that we know increase the risk of heart disease. (See chapter 13 on diet for details.) They are found in nearly all processed foods, including chips, baked goods, and prepared frozen foods.

The biggest problem with the saturated fat found in nonorganic meat is that it contains two classes of substances dangerous to the prostate: pesticides and estrogen-like drugs used to fatten livestock for market. High concentration of pesticides accumulate and rest in *our* fatty tissues, and increase our risk of cancer. Residues of synthetic estrogens in estrogen-like drugs used on livestock can have toxic effects on human tissues, even in minute amounts.

I'm not going to suggest that you get fanatical about never eating nonorganic meat, but I would certainly suggest that you find a reliable source of pesticide-free and hormone-free meat. If you have no local organic source, you'll find mail-order sources listed in the back of this book.

NUTRITIONAL APPROACHES TO PREVENTING AND STOPPING PROSTATE CANCER

My Eight Steps to Staying Power for Life are intended to preserve youth, prevent disease, and create a foundation for a healthy prostate. If you and your man work toward achieving a healthier lifestyle, you will also reduce your family's risk of all cancers, including prostate cancer.

Studies of specific nutrients and how they relate to prostate cancer risk reveal that zinc and vitamin D may be protective. Foods such as tomatoes, which contain *lycopene,* a carotenoid nutrient, are especially beneficial.

Linus Pauling, Nobel laureate biochemist and champion of the use of megadoses of vitamin C to prevent and cure many ills, co-authored *Cancer and Vitamin C* (published by The Linus Pauling Institute of

Science and Medicine in 1979). Dozens of studies and case histories are cited in which immune system activation with sodium ascorbate (buffered vitamin C) brought about reversals of cancer.

In studies of vitamin E and beta-carotene, these antioxidants have been found to inhibit the growth of prostate cancer cells. However, the effects of specific antioxidant nutrients on prostate cancer is much less consistent than on other cancers, giving us a clue that these cancers are probably largely hormone-driven.

If you follow the diet and supplement program I recommend in chapter 13, you and your family will get all of the above nutrients and more.

The Eight Steps take care to maintain a healthful balance that's less likely to promote out-of-control cell growth, even if a person's body has a few stray cancerous cells. Our immune systems can do away with a few cancerous cells here and there if we take good care of ourselves.

9

Keeping His Hair on His Head

In our modern, youth-craving culture, baldness is not an honored symbol of wisdom gained with passing years. Many balding men are viewed by themselves and others as less attractive and less virile than their hair-sporting counterparts. Hair loss seriously threatens the confidence of some men, and no remedy—be it a salve, a drug, a magical scalp tonic, artificial hair, or a surgical procedure—escapes their attention. Men spend billions of dollars and hours of valuable time every year in their quest to eradicate bald spots. I hope to see the day when balding is looked upon with something other than dread—perhaps simply as a natural change in the appearance of some men, like the arrival of facial hair with puberty and the graying of hair with advancing age. Until that day comes, the average balding man's interest in safe and permanent ways to keep his hair on his head is understandable.

Here are some of the available solutions to the problem of male pattern baldness (also called *androgenetic alopecia*). I'll talk about possible causes, the efficacy of available treatments, and what a man can do to keep his hair and scalp healthy.

WHAT CAUSES MALE PATTERN BALDNESS?

If we truly understood how male pattern baldness (MPG) occurs, you can be sure there would be a drug you could take to prevent it, but at the time of this writing there is no drug available that really prevents or reverses balding. However, we do know quite a bit, and there is a lot a man can do to slow the loss of hair.

By the age of forty, two-thirds of Caucasian men have lost noticeable amounts of hair. Hair loss can be the result of a number of factors, including medications, vitamin deficiencies, vitamin overdoses (particularly vitamin A), illnesses, and hormone imbalances. Some researchers have suggested that losing hair from the top of the head is a compensation for the growth of beard hairs, so that heat can escape from the scalp rather than the face! (Don't let him run to the bathroom and shave off his beard to save his scalp hair; the study found no difference in heat retention between shaved and grown-out beards.)

I'm going to focus on male pattern baldness, the kind of hair loss that affects up to 50 percent of men and is believed to be largely due to a combination of hormones and heredity.

Some men start to go bald in their early twenties, while others keep their hair until they hit andropause. There are those who begin to lose hair early, stop losing it for a few decades, and then begin to lose it again later in life. The typical pattern of hair loss starts at the hairline, with the edges receding to form an "M" shape. The top points of the "M" meet on the crown of the head; some hair may remain in the center of the forehead. Hair begins to be lost from the back of the head as well, and any remaining hair on the top of the head goes, leaving the characteristic horseshoe-shaped ring of hair around the sides and back of the head. In some cases, balding starts on the back of the head without recession of the hairline, and the bald spot moves forward. Remaining hair tends to be thinner and oilier.

If hair loss doesn't occur in either of these patterns, or if it occurs very quickly with large chunks of hair falling out at a time, it's probably not MPB. There might be a treatable cause.

Often, loss of hair from the scalp is accompanied by an alarming increase in hair growth on other parts of the body: the back, chest, belly, and even the ears and nose. Rotary nose-and-ear hair clippers designed to deal with the overgrowth in these areas can be easily obtained in department stores or from mail-order catalogs. Proper hormone balance should be able to minimize the growth of excess body hair. Laser hair removal can take care of excess growth as well—see chapter 10, "Laser Surgery Isn't Just for Women."

SOME HAIR AND SCALP ANATOMY

Hair follicles cover the scalp and much of the rest of the body and form pouches from which hairs sprout. Hairs grow from *root bulbs* that lie within the follicles. These tufts of live tissue enclose the living hair root and supply it with *keratin,* the protein needed to build the hair shaft. Each follicle also contains its own *sebaceous gland,* which secretes oily *sebum* into the follicle. Sebum lubricates hair and inhibits the growth of bacteria.

Each scalp hair has a growth phase that lasts for two to six years. The root bulbs are each supplied with fresh blood and nutrients by a single capillary. At the end of the growth phase, the root becomes inactive, and the hair and root bulb detach from the follicle. When a new hair begins to grow, it pushes the dead one out ahead of it, and with brushing or washing the old hair falls out.

It's normal to shed anywhere from twenty to a hundred and fifty hairs each day. On a balding scalp, the hairs that are lost are not replaced as quickly, and in balding areas the replacement hairs are very fine and pale. Many of the follicles on a balding scalp are healthy and have adequate circulation, but shrink, for reasons no one has been able to explain adequately. The sebaceous glands continue to produce oil in each follicle, with or without hair, which causes remaining hair and the bald scalp to be oilier.

The Hormone Connection

I talked about dihydrotestosterone (DHT), one of the derivatives of testosterone, in chapter 8. DHT is formed in various sites in our bodies by an enzyme called 5-alpha-reductase. Whereas testosterone regulates the development of secondary sex characteristics (deepening the voice, developing muscle, making sperm, and growing body hair), dihydrotestosterone regulates the development and growth of the prostate, penis, and testicles, as well as the pattern of facial, body, and scalp hair growth. DHT is produced in especially high concentrations in the prostate, adrenal glands, and scalp. Production of DHT doesn't appear to increase or decrease with age, but the sensitivity of the prostate and the hair follicles on the scalp and over the rest of the body to the influence of DHT does increase with passing years.

The hair follicles get a double whammy of DHT, because they each make their own within the hair follicles and are also exposed to it in blood that circulates to the area. Most research puts the blame for male pattern baldness on some aspect of the action of DHT that causes the follicles to degrade slowly and lose function, either producing spindly, weak hairs or dying off completely and producing no hair at all. Hair around the sides and back of the head seems resistant to the effects of DHT, and that's why hair transplants work—the tiny patches of hair farmed from the back of the head and sewn onto bald-ing areas don't fall out.

DHT is believed to act on the cells (called *dermal papillae*) in the center of the hair follicle bulb, which is where hair is made. The der-mal papillae in balding areas of the scalp are smaller and don't grow as well as those in areas with plenty of healthy hair. The higher the num-ber of active binding sites for DHT in the hair follicles, the more likely hair loss is to occur. Androgen-binding sites in follicles of bald-ing areas have a much stronger affinity for DHT than do those still growing hair. Drugs that block the testosterone to DHT conversion, such as the 5-alpha-dehydrogenase inhibitor finasteride (Proscar, now marketed as the hair-regrowth drug Propecia), often has the side effect of causing hair regrowth on balding parts of the scalp, but it's very fine, thin hair that falls out shortly after the drug treatment stops.

MAYBE BEING BALD ISN'T SUCH A BAD THING, CONSIDERING THE ALTERNATIVE

Castration is the only surefire preventive for androgenetic alopecia! Men without testicles never go bald. Eunuchs with a family history of baldness, on the other hand, promptly go bald when given supple-mental testosterone. That's pretty solid evidence for the role of hor-mone balance.

Women don't go bald too often because their hormonal milieu counteracts the male hormones that activate MPB. The hair follicles of women contain significantly fewer receptors for androgens and less 5-alpha-reductase than do those of men, and much higher concentra-tions of the enzyme that converts the androgen androstenedione to es-trogens. Female pattern baldness does exist, but women don't lose as much hair as do men, and hair loss occurs diffusely instead of in the distinctive pattern seen in men.

If one or both of a man's parents has hair loss, his chances are high of also losing hair. We don't yet know exactly what the connection is between the chromosomes and the actual hair loss. It may be that the gene for baldness increases the sensitivity of the hair follicles to DHT, or it may cause an increase in the number of DHT receptors in the follicles as a man ages.

BLOCKING DHT PRODUCTION NATURALLY

There are some natural approaches that will block the deleterious effects of DHT on hair follicles. Saw palmetto and zinc, both of which I highly recommend for prostate health, reduce the formation of DHT by inhibiting 5-alpha-reductase. Oral zinc and saw palmetto can cut down on the scalp's DHT load enough to slow hair loss. He should try 160 milligrams of saw palmetto and 15 to 30 milligrams of zinc picolinate twice a day, with 50 milligrams of B$_6$ every day.

I have also heard reports from men using natural progesterone cream for prostate enlargement that their hair stopped falling out. To try this, have him use about 1/8 teaspoon per day of a cream that contains 400 milligrams of progesterone per ounce. I do not recommend oral progesterone. (See chapter 8 for more details on progesterone.)

EXCESS SEBUM

The results of the work of a Japanese research team, headed by Dr. Yoshikata Inaba, point to excessive sebum production in the hair follicles as a major contributing factor in male pattern baldness. Excess sebum traps DHT in the hair follicle, allowing it more time to act on the root bulb. Oxidized fatty acids, which are always harmful to surrounding tissues, are also trapped inside the follicle when sebum is overproduced. According to some experts, when scalp pores become clogged with excess sebum, the hair root becomes malnourished.

Scientists who subscribe to this theory advise balding men to wash their hair often to cut down levels of surface sebum. Seborrheic dermatitis, a disorder that can cause flaking and itching of scalp skin; oily or dry scalp skin and hair; and acne, blackheads, whiteheads, or small red bumps around the hairline; can be a cause of excess sebum production.

Shampoos specifically designed for those who are losing their hair are formulated to decrease inflammation, clear away excess sebum, and nourish hair roots. Some are sold with solutions containing amino acids, special carbohydrates, and antioxidants, to be applied after shampooing. There are many to choose from, and a dermatologist can tell you which ones are best. Keeping the scalp clean and well nourished is an important part of any hair-maintenance program.

THE HEART DISEASE CONNECTION

Men who bald significantly before the age of fifty-five have a slightly higher risk of dying of heart disease. DHT levels tend to be *lower* in men with heart disease, so this connection leads us away from looking at hormonal causes. Could the atrophy of hair follicles be due in part to poor scalp circulation?

A tendency toward clogged blood vessels means damage to the arteries that feed the heart muscle, and also to the tiny capillary networks that feed the whole body on a cellular level. Decreased capillary circulation to scalp skin could decrease the function of hair follicles over a period of years. Without adequate blood flow, follicles atrophy and can't nourish the root bulb. Increase in scalp circulation appears to be the mechanism by which minoxidil (Rogaine), the best-selling baldness remedy, regrows hair. Other products are available that should improve scalp circulation through stimulation of the nitric oxide system within the blood vessels. Talk to your pharmacist for the best one.

Scalp circulation can be improved by eating well, exercising, and taking circulation-enhancing supplements. (I'll go into more detail about the circulatory system in chapter 12, "Resisting the Diseases and Debilities of Aging.") Another approach to try is scalp massage: Turn the head upside down by squatting or sitting and bending forward at the waist, and massage the scalp skin with all ten fingers.

Rub in small circles, applying enough pressure to move the skin around. Just inverting the head for five to fifteen minutes per day will increase blood flow to the scalp. Inverted poses in yoga can reverse the pull of gravity and send plenty of freshly oxygenated blood up to the head. Brushing hair from the roots twice to three times daily stimulates circulation to the roots and encourages empty follicles to sprout healthy new hairs.

HYPOTHYROIDISM

Hypothyroidism, in which the thyroid gland produces insufficient amounts of its hormones, is a major cause of hair loss. It's estimated that around 25 percent of Americans are slightly deficient in this essential metabolic regulator, and the slightest disregulation in thyroid hormone production can have widespread effects.

Indications that a man might be low on thyroid hormone include losing hair; feeling lethargic; often feeling cold; unexplained weight gain; dry, scaly skin; hair like straw; ridges on the fingernails; or experiencing a loss of libido that's not remedied by other aspects of this program. A doctor can test for low thyroid hormone levels and, if necessary, add it to the hormone replacement regimen.

Raw brassica vegetables (Brussels sprouts, cauliflower, broccoli, kale, watercress, soybeans, peanuts, cabbage) contain goitrogens, which block the thyroid gland's ability to function properly. These vegetables and legumes should always be cooked before eating. Overexposure to chlorine and fluoride can also block thyroid hormone production. This is one of many good reasons to have a high-quality water filter installed in your kitchen and to fight to keep fluoride out of your community's water system.

Specific nutrients are needed for the manufacture of thyroid hormones. The mineral iodine is found in sea vegetables and iodized salt. A high-potency B complex supplement supports thyroid function as well.

INFLAMMATION AND FREE RADICALS
PLAY A ROLE HERE, TOO

Researchers are also finding that an inflammatory process is taking place in hair follicles on balding scalp. The body's own immune factors begin to infiltrate the root bulb, affecting the ability of stem cells to do their work. As the root bulb dies, more immune cells move in to clean up the debris. There may be a connection to infections caused by increased sebum production and clogging of the follicle, with the immune response to the infection starting the inflammatory cascade that results in hair loss.

It's also possible that free radical damage plays a role in male pattern baldness. Levels of the endogenous (made in the body) antioxidant glutathione are measurably lower in sebaceous glands of balding areas of the scalp, and the level of the enzyme that activates glutathione is very high. This indicates that the free radical–scavenging capacity of glutathione is being depleted by excessive free radical formation. Follow the recommendations in chapter 5, "Keeping Cells Young by Squelching Oxidation." Have him eat plenty of garlic, asparagus, and a few eggs a week to keep glutathione levels high (these foods contain sulfur, a mineral needed for the production of glutathione). Remember, too, that there are shampoos available that contain antioxidants and amino acids. Ask a dermatologist or hairstylist for recommendations, or shop around on the Internet.

NO MAGIC BULLETS

It's unlikely that any one of these possible causes of baldness is the sole cause of the problem. A combination of several factors—including heredity, changing hormone levels, clogging from excess sebum, increased hair follicle sensitivity to hormones, poor scalp circulation, inflammation, and oxidative stress—is most likely to blame. Cause-and-effect relationships probably exist among these factors. For example, DHT can be trapped in the follicles by excess sebum, and sluggish circulation can lead to increased free radical formation. Some factors have greater effects on some men than on others.

SUMMARY OF NUTRIENTS FOR HEALTHY HAIR AND SCALP

Good nutrition is as important for hair and scalp health as it is for the health of the rest of the body. Many of the essential nutrients are already a part of the supplement program, so don't be daunted by this list.

- Eat fresh fish and sea vegetables such as kelp, dulse, and nori a couple of times a week. These are rich sources of iodine, needed for the manufacture of thyroid hormones.
- Take vitamins E, A, and C as recommended in chapter 5 on oxidation.
- Take B complex vitamins, especially folic acid, biotin, inositol, and PABA (para-amino-benzoic acid), as recommended in my multivitamin guidelines.
- Take minerals: silica, magnesium, calcium, selenium, potassium, and phosphorus. Some vitamin formulations contain all these minerals specifically for hair health. The supplement program I've outlined should give adequate amounts of all but silica. Apples, avocados, honey, and nuts are rich in silica. Eating several servings of fruits and vegetables and some lean chicken or fish each day is a good way to get sufficient minerals.
- Follow the recommendations on circulation (pages 218–219) to keep scalp blood vessels healthy.

PRESCRIPTION DRUGS FOR MPB

When researchers first tested minoxidil in 1988, they were hoping to add it to the arsenal of powerful prescription drugs on the market for hypertension. They found that it did lower blood pressure, but with a curious and common side effect: it caused subjects to grow hair on their heads, backs, eyebrows, arms, and legs. The pharmaceutical giant Upjohn raced through testing of topical minoxidil as a baldness remedy and soon launched an aggressive marketing campaign focused on America's twenty-million-plus balding men. In their advertising, Upjohn claims that Rogaine causes moderate hair growth in 25 percent of users after four months, and moderate to dense growth in 50 percent of users with a year's steady use. Impartial medical researchers come up with some less encouraging figures, saying that 8 percent at four months and about 40 percent at one year is more accurate. To have any success at all, Rogaine users must apply the solution to balding areas twice a day for at least four months, and it must be continued indefinitely to maintain the new hair growth. Once Rogaine therapy is stopped, the hair falls out again. It's also expensive, costing $600 to $1,000 a year.

The people who have the best results with Rogaine have small balding areas, ten centimeters or less across, and have been balding for less than ten years. They are in their twenties or thirties and are not balding at the temples, as the drug seems to work better on the top and back of the scalp than on receding hairline. Side effects include skin irritation, itching, prickling, headache, dizzy spells, and (rarely) irregularities in heart rhythm. Because even topical medications are absorbed into the general circulation, Rogaine isn't a good idea for anyone with a history of irregular heartbeats or heart disease. It used to be available only by prescription, but now is sold over the counter.

No one is certain how Rogaine works to grow hair and stop hair loss. It has potent *vasodilating* (blood vessel expanding) effects, which is why researchers originally thought it would be a good high blood pressure drug. There are plenty of vasodilating drugs on the market that don't grow hair, however. The best guess is that minoxidil delays hair from falling out and prompts new growth by stimulating the root bulb.

Because balding isn't dangerous to any part of the body besides the ego, it doesn't make sense to bombard a system with powerful drugs just to regrow hair. This can disrupt the body's delicate balance and cause more trouble in the long run than it's worth.

Finasteride is a 5-alpha-reductase inhibitor, commonly prescribed to men with benign prostatic hyperplasia (BPH). It blocks the transformation of testosterone to dihydrotestosterone (DHT), and often has the side effect of partially reversing male pattern baldness. In a study by Merck, the manufacturer of Propecia, 86 percent of 1,500 balding men ages 18 to 41 who started on a regimen of oral finasteride stopped losing their hair, and some even grew significant amounts of new hair. Propecia works best for men in the very early stages of hair loss. Balding on the top and back of the head responds better to treatment, which for the most part halts future hair loss rather than restoring hair already lost. Theoretically, saw palmetto should have a similar effect.

SURGICAL SOLUTIONS

If a man has the gene for baldness, he may be able to slow hair loss, but there's very little hope of stopping it completely without surgery.

The process of *hair transplantation* takes a lot of time and money, averaging one to four sessions (the less hair he's lost, the fewer sessions he'll need) at about $12,000 per session. Health insurance doesn't cover the procedure, no matter how much psychological trauma hair loss is causing. Still, a quarter of a million American men have hair transplants each year.

The surgeon removes tiny patches of hair, an eighth of an inch around, from the healthy, dense-growth area on the back of the head, and places them in front of the receding hairline. Techniques have been developed that make grafts look more natural; smaller grafts are strategically placed to soften the "plug" appearance at the hairline. The implantation of these micro- and minigrafts (1 to 4 hairs apiece) can require extra sessions and more money.

Right after surgery, scabs form. The hairs fall out and are soon replaced by new, permanent hairs. If Rogaine therapy is started within a couple of days after surgery, the transplanted hairs don't fall out.

Hair transplantation works best in men with hair loss only on the front of the scalp, and who don't expect to lose too much more hair (look at his dad or his mother's father to see into his scalp's future). Other procedures, including scalp reduction, flaps, or tissue expansion, might be needed to complete the effect of a full head of hair in some men.

Scalp reduction (galeoplasty) is intended for men with visible bald spots no more than three inches across on the crown of the head. A section of bald scalp is removed and the edges are pulled up and sewn together. Small grafts are used to fill in gaps. Galeoplasty costs about $1,600 per surgery, and if the bald area is large, more than one surgery is necessary.

In a *flap* procedure, a large piece of scalp is detached at one end from a hair-bearing area, and the free end is brought over the bald area in the front and sewn down. This tends to look artificial, and needs extra micrografts to soften the resulting straight hairline.

In *tissue expansion,* silicone bags are implanted beneath scalp areas with hair, and saline solution is added to gradually expand them over a period of a few weeks. Once the skin is stretched out, the bags are removed and a scalp reduction is performed. If a man is free of heart disease and diabetes, and likes to wear hats large enough to camouflage the strange appearance of expanding balloons beneath his scalp, he can have this procedure done for around $4,000.

If your man is interested in surgery, be forewarned that even the best surgeon might not be able to make a new head of hair look natural. Try to get a referral from a satisfied friend, or write or call the American Academy of Facial Plastic and Reconstructive Surgery (1110 Vermont Avenue NW, Suite 220, Washington, DC 20005; 1-800-332-3223) to get a list of credentialed surgeons.

ANSWERS FOR MALE PATTERN BALDNESS

As is the case with any physiological process, the causes, effects, and remedies are multifactorial. A comprehensive approach works much better than any "magic bullet."

10

Laser Surgery Isn't Just for Women

Although looks aren't everything, they're certainly part and parcel of self-image and success. It used to be that fashion magazines, cosmetics, weight control, and plastic surgery were concerns only of women. Men's magazines now focus on these topics as well, and products to address these issues are pitched to men.

Aging causes changes in the skin that were once thought to be irreversible. With the advent of processes like dermabrasion (a wire brush is used to buff damaged skin away) and chemical peels (acid is used to burn off top layers of skin), dermatologists and plastic surgeons found that they could take a decade or more off patients' faces without giving them face-lifts. Now the amazing technology of lasers is allowing doctors to use light to literally erase fine wrinkles and under-eye bags, permanently get rid of scars, semi-permanently get rid of unwanted body hair, and even treat skin cancers and warts.

I do laser surgery in my practice, and I know it works. In this chapter we'll cover all the information needed to make a decision about whether laser skin resurfacing or other cosmetic laser procedures are appropriate, including how to pick a competent surgeon and exactly what to expect before, during, and after the procedure.

SKIN AGING

Collagen fibers create a flexible meshwork over which our skin cells are stretched. As we age, these fibers actually increase in number and their bonds become tighter. Stretchy *elastin* fibers form cross-linkages that pull skin into folds as years creep by. The *ground substance* that makes up the cellular "cement" between collagen and elastin fibers becomes less fluid and more like, well, cement. Nutrients and oxygen are less able to travel from cell to cell as this meshwork of structural proteins becomes tangled. Skin cells die off as a result.

We know that avoiding excess sun exposure is an important way to slow down skin aging. Ultraviolet rays hitting the skin cause oxidation of skin cells and underlying tissues, and anyone who insists on keeping the body and face darkly tanned can expect to have quite a few more wrinkles and age spots than his palefaced counterparts.

Just in case the man in your life isn't convinced that he should take supplements, eat well, and drink plenty of water, he should know that doing so will also benefit the appearance of his skin. Creams for the face and body containing antioxidants are a good bet; the nutrients scavenge free radicals as they form. Exercise that brings up a good sweat is a terrific skin conditioner—it brings plentiful blood flow to the skin's surface. Facial massage is another great rejuvenator of tired skin. Hormone replacement, particularly growth hormone, will almost certainly take years off his complexion.

When all else fails and the ravages of time have taken enough of a toll to make him not want to look in the mirror, he might want to consider laser skin resurfacing.

WHAT EXACTLY IS LASER SKIN RESURFACING?

A *laser* is a very intense, pulsating light beam. LASER is actually an acronym that stands for *Light Amplification by the Stimulated Emission of Radiation.* Several different kinds of lasers are used in medicine: as scalpels to make incisions, as cauterizers to seal blood vessels closed, or to selectively burn away thin layers of skin. (See Table 10.1.) Each use requires a beam containing a specific wavelength of light. Lasers can literally vaporize tissues, which makes them useful for tasks like removing hair, warts, varicose veins, and tumors—and for smoothing hard-earned wrinkles.

The goal of the surgeon is to remove the aged outer layer of skin and stimulate the formation of new, tauter skin in its place. At lower intensities, the laser can be used to diminish individual wrinkles. Fine, shallow lines are the best kinds to treat with lasers.

After laser treatment, skin is stimulated to produce new collagen and elastin fibers. The end result is a smoother, younger-looking complexion that should stay that way for at least a few years with proper care.

Lasers are precise instruments that allow the surgeon to specifically "zap" certain areas. Results are usually superior to other kinds of skin resurfacing procedures, and the risk of infection is much lower because there's no breaking of the skin's surface. Laser treatment greatly reduces the risk of scarring and skin pigment changes and decreases recovery time, compared with older methods of skin resurfacing.

People between the ages of 35 and 60 are more likely to have good results. Someone who is older and doesn't have a lot of deep wrinkles can still expect good results. Medium-toned Caucasian skin that doesn't scar easily responds best to this type of plastic surgery.

Patients are given local anesthesia if they're just having the laser treatment. For other surgical procedures done at the same time, they'll probably have general anesthesia. The laser treatment itself is relatively brief, depending on how much detailed work is being done.

The patient should plan to take a day or two off after the surgery. His face will be swollen, sore, bright red, oozing, and itchy. It takes at least a week for the skin to grow back. People vary in the time required to heal completely, but it shouldn't be more than a couple of weeks until the swelling is gone. Cosmetics should cover residual redness. The skin may be swollen and have a reddish cast for up to six months after the procedure.

It's absolutely essential to wear broad-brimmed hats or stay in the shade for at least six months after laser surgery. Those who don't are likely to develop blotchy discolorations *(hyperpigmentation)* that will require additional treatments. Even being careful about sun exposure, the chances of developing hyperpigmentation are pretty good—20 to 30 percent of those who undergo laser skin resurfacing end up with this side effect. Most surgeons have their patients pretreat their facial skin with bleaching cream for two weeks before and three weeks after surgery. This usually takes care of the problem.

OTHER USES FOR COSMETIC LASER SURGERY

Visible Blood Vessels
Enlarged facial blood vessels, usually on the nose, are a common cosmetic complaint. Special kinds of lasers can seal off these vessels so that they disintegrate; they are then reabsorbed by the body.

Laser Hair Removal

Many andropausal men are the butt of jokes having to do with hair loss from the head and hair growth in spots where it doesn't belong. If balancing hormones doesn't stop the growth of coarse hair on the back and neck, the unwanted hair can be removed with a quick, easy laser procedure. Certain lasers are used to target hair follicles, injuring them so that hairs fall out. The follicles do recover, but it can take many months before hair sprouts again.

Laser Tooth Whitening

Years of exposure to coffee, tea, heavily fluoridated water, or cigarette smoke, or long-term treatment with the antibiotic tetracycline, can discolor teeth. Lasers are the newest, fastest way to have teeth whitened. The dentist applies a hydrogen peroxide solution to teeth and zaps them with a laser beam, increasing the natural bleaching action of the hydrogen peroxide. Laser tooth whitening takes only two hours. It's completely painless and the results are immediate, with very little maintenance after it's over. The cost is about $900 and is not covered by insurance. To find out which dentists offer this procedure, ask your usual dentist. She may be able to do the procedure in her office.

Laser Blepharoplasty

With aging, the upper and lower eyelids can begin to sag and pockets of fat may form. Not only can this be unattractive, but it can impede vision. Lifting of droopy eyelids *(blepharoplasty)* has been done with a scalpel for years, and has taken years off the faces of many satisfied patients. Now blepharoplasty can be done with lasers. Using the laser has many advantages—less postoperative pain (because the laser seals off nerve endings as it cuts), shorter recovery period, less bleeding (because the laser beam seals off blood vessels as well), and less swelling and bruising after surgery. Lasers also sterilize the areas they cut—and that means reduced risk of infection.

This outpatient surgery is done under local anesthetic. The incisions made by the laser are sealed with small stitches, which are removed within five or six days. Ice packs are used on the eyes for the first day or two postoperatively, plus antibiotic eyedrops to prevent infection. The patient should recover completely within two weeks' time, but be prepared to take a couple of days off right after surgery and to wear dark glasses or cosmetics to conceal redness and swelling for the next week.

Other Skin Problems for the Laser

Tattoos, age spots, and scars can be removed, and skin cancers and warts can be eliminated, with different wavelengths of light.

WHAT ARE THE RISKS?

Any surgical procedure carries with it the risk of complications. In an evaluation of 500 patients who had laser skin resurfacing on 1,589 different sites, the most common complication was swelling. Every one of the patients studied had swollen faces for an average of four and a half months. Dark discolorations were seen in 37 percent of patients and were more common in darker-skinned individuals. Acne and dermatitis (rash) were seen in around 10 percent of cases, and 7.4 percent of patients had outbreaks of herpes simplex virus in the area treated, even though some had no previous history of the virus. Scarring, loss of skin pigment *(hypopigmentation),* and infections other than herpes virus were seen in less than 1 percent of these subjects.

HOW MUCH DOES IT COST?

On average, laser cosmetic surgery costs $3,000 to $5,000. Insurers won't pay for it, but some providers offer payment plans to patients. Hair removal can cost from $500 to $800, depending on the area.

Table 10.1 Lasers Used for Different Procedures

Carbon Dioxide (CO_2) laser	Skin resurfacing, scar removal, warts, skin cancers, darkly pigmented spots, tooth whitening
Erbium: YAG laser	Skin resurfacing
Argon laser	Removal of dark red discolorations and visible blood vessels (varicose veins)
Yellow light lasers	Removal of dark red discolorations and visible blood vessels (varicose veins)
Argon-pumped tunable dye lasers	Can produce yellow light; also can be "tuned" to produce red light for treatment of skin cancers
Copper vapor laser	Can produce yellow light; also can be "tuned" to produce green light to erase brown pigmented lesions like freckles and age spots
Long-pulsed ruby laser and long-pulsed alexandrite laser	Removal of unwanted body hair
Q-switched ruby laser and Q-switched alexandrite laser	Tattoo, freckle, age spot removal

Table 10.1 Lasers Used for Different Procedures (continued)

Q-switched neodymium: YAG laser	Can produce infrared light to remove dark tattoos and dark skin lesions, or can be "tuned" to produce green light for treatment of brown pigmented lesions like freckles and age spots; also used for hair removal
KTP laser	For treatment of red or brown discolorations

11

Keeping the Blood Vessels Clear and Strong

Heart disease is at the top of the list of diseases that kill men in Westernized countries. It takes its toll not only in terms of numbers of deaths, but also in the cost of care. Millions of medications, medical procedures, and surgeries are dispensed each year to try to prevent people at risk from suffering a fatal heart attack. I and my colleagues in the field of anti-aging medicine firmly believe modern medicine is missing the point. In the quest to *cure* heart disease with drug cocktails and bypass surgeries, too little energy has been focused on *prevention.*

In this chapter, I'll talk about causes, effects, and solutions for the prevention of heart disease, hypertension, and adult-onset diabetes, all of which are related in some way to poor circulatory health. I'll discuss a program that supports the health of men's blood vessels so they can avoid prescription drugs and surgery.

Disease of the arteries is the result of a certain set of conditions throughout the body. These conditions predispose the vessels to the kind of damage that disrupts blood flow. When this damage is going on in a man's blood vessels, he may receive signals from his body in the form of hypertension, less-than-ideal cholesterol counts, or adult-onset diabetes.

In the quest for a quick-fix, magic solution to the problem of artery disease, researchers have attempted to ferret out cause-and-effect relationships. When studies showed that high blood cholesterol levels had a link to greatly increased incidence of heart disease, the drug companies scrambled to produce and test cholesterol-lowering drugs. Diet experts extolled the virtues of a diet free of saturated fat and cholesterol. All the hype hit the public eye before there was prudent consideration of whether the high cholesterol was *causing* the heart disease or not. Now it's becoming clear that high blood cholesterol, in and of itself, doesn't cause arteries to clog.

The same thing has happened with high blood pressure. There's no contesting the fact that high blood pressure is very injurious to the blood vessels throughout the body, and that it needs to stay below certain levels. What's not so clear is whether the powerful drugs being used to treat hypertension are worth the price paid in side effects and long-term damage throughout the body. Those who use the drugs don't reap much benefit in the long run.

Blood cholesterol and blood pressure are kept at ideal levels by a number of feedback mechanisms. Neither of these tightly controlled and balanced systems goes out of balance without reason. Coronary artery disease and adult-onset diabetes are the consequences of years of an unhealthy lifestyle combined with a genetic predisposition for those diseases.

When our lifestyle choices lead to this situation, resetting of limits is the best the body can do under the circumstances. Blood pressure, insulin levels, and blood cholesterol are maintained at higher levels as the body attempts to deal with constant imbalance. The only solution that will work to eradicate coronary artery disease is one that brings the body back into balance.

HEART DISEASE

Heart disease is a lay term for *coronary artery disease,* also known as *coronary atherosclerosis.* Heart vessels are especially vulnerable to damage; they wrap tightly around the heart muscle, and are squeezed and yanked with each heartbeat. That's a lot of mechanical stress on the twists and turns of those vessels. Tiny tears happen frequently and attempts to repair them without the needed substances can cause blockages. Vessels in the brain, organs, and extremities are, to a lesser extent, affected by atherosclerosis. Here's what happens:

1. The walls of the blood vessels that bring oxygen and nutrients to the heart muscle are damaged. Specialized blood cells called platelets are drawn to the damaged area. This is the body's natural response to injury—the formation of a clot on an artery wall is similar to the formation of a scab over a cut. One of cholesterol's many roles in the body is in healing injuries to the blood vessels, and so it also adheres to the site of the injury.

2. The same imbalances that predisposed the vessel wall to injury promote an overblown healing response. Platelets and cholesterol molecules collect, the walls of the vessel in the area constrict (a response meant to lessen the shear of blood flow past the injury, but which can go overboard under these circumstances), and *growth factors* are secreted.

3. The growth factors attract more cells to the site, and the smooth muscle cells grow larger. White blood cells filled with cholesterol

(macrophages) stick to the area as well, and the cholesterol begins to infiltrate the walls of the vessels. Growth factors are secreted by the ever-expanding mass of cells, and connective tissue and calcium are incorporated to support the new tissue growth (*plaque* or *lesion*).

Plaques can grow very slowly and never cause a problem, or they may grow rapidly and compromise blood flow within a year of the initial vessel wall injury. Symptoms of plaque buildup can include angina pain from blocked heart vessels; memory loss; sudden, temporary loss of vision from blocked brain vessels; or shooting pains in the legs with activity, caused by blocked vessels to the legs. Chronically constricted arteries makes blockages more likely. Turbulent blood flow and cramping of artery walls also make the lesions more likely to tear or rupture, sending clots into the circulation, which can become lodged in other partially blocked vessels.

Heart attack, or *myocardial infarction,* describes the situation in which flow is completely cut off to a portion of the heart wall. This can happen if a blood clot forms and lodges in a clogged area, or by coronary vessels going into spasm. Even if you survive a heart attack—which is very likely these days because of medical technologies that allow quick unclogging of the affected vessel—a chunk of the wall of the heart may not, and that compromises the heart's ability to function.

Stroke, or *cerebrovascular accident,* is another common cause of debility in aging men. This occurs when a blood vessel in the brain becomes clogged or bursts.

Congestive heart failure happens when the heart muscle has been starved of oxygen for so long that it can't pump hard enough to get blood through the circulation. Fluid pools in the lungs and makes breathing difficult. On a smaller scale, the tiny capillaries that bring blood to each cell deteriorate when they don't receive sufficient blood flow from the larger vessels upstream. That means poor circulation in the smaller blood vessels as well, with microscopic damage to just about every organ in your body.

It isn't a pretty picture, but don't despair. There are plenty of ways to get blood vessels healthy so they can keep the heart, brain, organs, and limbs in tip-top shape.

Heart disease doesn't come from nowhere like a thief in the night. It isn't a random stroke of bad luck. A number of predisposing factors lead, after years and years, to that heart attack or stroke. Genetics is one of them. If a man's father or mother had heart disease, that's all the more reason for him to be taking as many preventive measures as are available.

We all know that if we don't exercise and eat a healthy diet, our risk of heart disease rises sharply. Hypertension, diabetes, and high cholesterol also create an increased risk. That's the basic picture. But what about all the other so-called "risk factors" we've been told about, like eating too much cholesterol or saturated fat? Just what comprises a "heart-healthy diet"? How about sugar? Does having a stressful life really make us more susceptible? Does taking certain vitamins really reduce our risk?

There are many questions and answers, and the sheer bulk of information can be dizzying to sift through. I'd like to try to make it simple by talking about the most basic causes of blood vessel disease. A grasp of the imbalances that cause blood vessel health to deteriorate shows how the solutions work. Even if the man in your life already has high blood pressure or high cholesterol, or if he's already had heart surgery, applying this knowledge can prevent the problem from worsening or recurring, and it can even eradicate it altogether.

Diseased arteries aren't caused by any one thing. That's why pharmaceutical "magic bullets" or isolated changes in lifestyle don't work to prevent them. Oscar, a college buddy of mine, figured that he could live on potato chips, pizza, and beer as long as he went for a run every day—and he ended up on the operating table having a four-way bypass.

COMMON DENOMINATORS

For the sake of clarity and conciseness, I'll break down the research on the causes of artery disease to its important common denominators—elements that knock the system out of balance. That imbalance manifests as high blood pressure, high cholesterol, and even diabetes, with artery disease not far behind. Controlling these few factors with the right lifestyle manipulations can prevent a heart attack and several of the other diseases that tend to occur due to the same factors—like peripheral vascular disease, stroke, congestive heart failure, and *multi-infarct dementia,* in which clogs in the tiny blood vessels throughout the brain cause a series of small strokes that can go unnoticed, but result in memory loss and deteriorating brain function.

WHAT DAMAGES THE LINING (ENDOTHELIUM) OF THE BLOOD VESSELS

Substances that damage the blood vessels include excess oxidized cholesterol, chronic high levels of insulin *(hyperinsulinemia),* deficiency of vitamin C, and too much of an amino acid called *homocysteine* in the bloodstream. All of these have a tendency to slash tiny holes in the linings of arteries. Plaques form as the body's healing systems try to fix the injury.

Remember from the chapter on oxidation that when free radicals are formed, they can grab onto proteins, DNA, cholesterol, and fats and oxidize them. At that point, the newly oxidized molecules begin to damage surrounding tissues. Lipoprotein molecules are our cholesterol transporters, carrying cholesterol to where it's needed. LDL (low-density lipoprotein) is specifically designed to deposit cholesterol where blood vessel injury has occurred. This healing mechanism goes haywire when there's rampant injury and high levels of circulating LDL. Low-density lipoprotein cholesterol is also particularly vulnerable to oxidation. Depositing oxidized LDL on your arteries is a one-way street to heart disease. Thus, you can understand why high LDL cholesterol doesn't cause heart disease per se: it's the body's healing response to an injury. And that is why cholesterol-lowering drugs don't heal heart disease: they only suppress a symptom of heart disease, while the causes go on unchecked.

LDL cholesterol can also be overoxidized by excess heavy metals. An overload of lead, iron, copper, and mercury creates an ideal environment for the oxidation of LDL. We also consume a lot of oxidized (unsaturated) fats in our standard American diet—few people go a single day without eating something that's been cooked at high temperatures in a polyunsaturated fat. Unstable fats can become oxidized just from being left out at room temperature. Even healthy unsaturated oils like fish oil can easily become oxidized. Oxidized fats float through the circulation and cause all kinds of damage to blood vessel linings; they then can become part of the plaques themselves. (See chapter 13 for details on good and bad fats.) This is one of the reasons that I don't recommend large daily amounts of flax oil or other unsaturated oils. They can have health benefits in small amounts, but over the long term, they contribute heavily to the oxidation load in the body.

DIABETES

Diabetes is a disease that directly harms the blood vessels, with tragic consequences.

Adult-onset diabetes, also known as Type 2 or non–insulin-dependent diabetes mellitus (NIDDM), is caused by a lifetime of eating mostly processed foods rich in bad fats and sugars, combined with little exercise. Although diabetes isn't in itself a disease of the blood vessels, it is a major cause of blood vessel disease throughout the body. Diabetic men are two to three times more likely to suffer heart attacks, stroke, and peripheral vascular disease. Deterioration of the capillary networks that feed the eyes causes vision loss in many diabetics.

When adult-onset diabetes sets in, changes occur in the cells' ability to use insulin. Insulin's job is to transport glucose out of the blood-stream and into the cells so that it can be used for energy. It also sup-ports the storage of excess calories as fat. For reasons still not well understood (but almost always associated with obesity), cells stop let-ting glucose in, no matter how much insulin the pancreas pumps out. Something prevents insulin and body cells from understanding each other's language, so that insulin and glucose levels in the bloodstream become elevated. Fats and proteins become the only accessible fuels. We can survive that way for some time, because the liver can make glucose (sugar) from proteins, but the person who experiences hyper-insulinemia (high blood insulin levels) and hyperglycemia (high blood sugar levels) doesn't feel well at all. Symptoms include fatigue, unex-plained weight loss, very frequent urination, and unquenchable thirst. Blood fats rise precipitously. Untreated diabetics can become danger-ously *ketotic,* a state in which the by-products of fat metabolism build up and acidify the body. Severe, unchecked ketosis leads to coma and even death.

If the diabetes isn't controlled, the pancreas, which has been strug-gling to pump out more and more insulin to try to fill the need for sugars in the cells, eventually becomes exhausted and stops making in-sulin. At that point, supplemental injections of insulin become neces-sary for survival.

This cascade of events seems to have something to do with weight gain, because adult-onset diabetes occurs almost exclusively in over-weight people. Weight loss invariably improves glucose uptake in peo-ple whose insulin hasn't been working well. Those who tend to gain the pounds on their midsections are most likely to develop diabetes in their later years. Insulin resistance may be the body's way of prevent-ing further weight gain. The body is saying, in effect, "All right, you've had ample nourishment, and you've got all this extra fat stored up. Don't use the carbohydrates until you use up all that energy stored in the fat!"

Insulin, in too-high concentrations, is extremely harmful to blood vessel walls. Chronically high blood sugars are also very damaging. Adult-onset diabetes is epidemic these days. Millions are on their way to full-blown diabetes and don't know it. A simple glucose tolerance test at a doctor's office can show whether insulin levels are above ideal levels. If they are, it's essential to take action now—because blood vessels are being ravaged every day that he doesn't.

Virtually all Type 2 diabetes can be well controlled through diet, exercise, and good nutritional supplementation. For details, please read *Prescription Alternatives* by Earl Mindell, R.Ph., Ph.D., and Virginia Hopkins, and for good dietary advice, read *Protein Power* by Michael and Mary Dan Eades, M.D.s.

HOMOCYSTEINE

Homocysteine is an amino acid that is created in the body by the breakdown of methionine, another amino acid. However, it is toxic in too-high concentrations. Meats and dairy products are rich in methionine. In a healthy body, homocysteine is quickly transformed back into methionine or broken down into cysteine, an amino acid with many important functions. Cysteine helps to draw excess copper out of the body, helps protect us from toxins, and is converted into the powerful antioxidant glutathione. The N-acetyl cysteine (NAC) form is itself an important antioxidant.

Folate, vitamin B_6, vitamin B_{12}, and a substance secreted from the stomach lining called *intrinsic factor* (necessary for the absorption of B vitamins) are all needed to make these transformations. When we are deficient in these nutrients—and many Americans are—we can't process homocysteine fast enough. It accumulates and damages our blood vessel walls.

Recent large-scale studies have shown a very strong association between homocysteine levels in the blood and risk of heart attack. One study from the *Journal of the American Medical Association* showed that only a 12 percent increase in homocysteine levels raised heart attack risk 3.4 times!

VITAMIN C

Vitamin C is a necessary component of collagen, the "glue" that holds artery walls together. Without vitamin C in the diet, blood vessels deteriorate and become leaky. In the days when sailors fell prey to scurvy, they died of massive internal bleeding as blood vessels literally dissolved for lack of vitamin C. In one study of 1,605 Finnish men, the risk of heart attack was 3.5 times greater in those with the lowest vitamin C levels. Matthias Rath, M.D., one of our foremost researchers of the nutrition–heart disease connection, believes that atherosclerosis is in part the body's attempt to lay down cellular cement to keep blood vessel walls from becoming leaky. Yet another reason to take vitamin C every day!

RX FOR ARTERY DAMAGE

Antioxidant nutrients are the most powerful weapons against artery damage caused by oxidation. Vitamins C and E both protect against oxidation; try 400 IU of E and 2,000 milligrams of C every day in divided doses. The trace mineral selenium helps vitamin E do its work, so be sure there's 200 micrograms in his daily multivitamin. (If you're following my vitamin guidelines he should be getting these amounts of vitamins every day.) Refer to chapter 5, "Keeping Cells Young by Squelching Oxidation," for general guidelines on antioxidant protection.

Recent studies reveal the protective effects of *flavonoids* against heart disease as well. Flavonoids are compounds found in whole foods like fruits, vegetables, nuts, and seeds, as well as in flowers, leaves, and bark, in association with vitamin C. In a large study done in the Netherlands on subjects ages sixty-five to eighty-four, those who took in the most flavonoids had a one-third lower risk of cardiovascular disease than those who took in the least amount of bioflavonoids. Flavonoids effectively scavenge free radicals and protect vitamin E from being oxidized (remember that when an antioxidant neutralizes a free radical, it momentarily becomes oxidized itself and needs to be renewed by other antioxidants). Some flavonoids are found in grape-seed extract, green tea, and quercetin, all of which can be obtained through supplements.

The herbs ginkgo biloba and bilberry extract both contain potent protectors of LDL. He can take 320 milligrams of ginkgo biloba and 500 milligrams of mixed flavonoids per day.

Avoid oxidized or very unstable fats whenever possible. Fried foods are generally a bad idea, but if he absolutely must have them, fry them in a more stable saturated fat like butter, lard, or coconut oil. (Instead of potato chips or french fries, try this: Thinly slice potatoes or yams. Brush them with some extra-virgin olive oil. Sprinkle on some sea salt, and bake the slices on a cookie sheet until crisp.) Please stay completely away from unsaturated oils such as corn oil and soy oil, as well as partially hydrogenated vegetable oils. Use mostly olive and canola oils for cooking. (See chapter 13 for details.)

Supplement all the B vitamins to bring homocysteine concentrations down to safe levels. He can take a B complex with each meal if his multivitamin doesn't contain adequate amounts. (See chapter 14 for amounts of B vitamins to take daily.)

RX FOR BLOOD SUGAR CONTROL

To control insulin levels, start with a diet low in processed carbohydrates (which include white flour, white rice, pasta, and chips) and sugars. Eat balanced meals that include fresh vegetables, protein foods, healthy fats, and complex carbohydrates such as whole grains, legumes, or brown rice.

Men who want to avoid diabetes should get some daily exercise. Exercise dramatically improves glucose uptake in diabetics, which means lowered blood sugars and insulin levels.

Diabetics must check their blood sugars four times a day and keep them strictly within limits prescribed by a doctor.

Since diabetics tend to be deficient in certain nutrients, supplements often improve blood sugar levels. I suggest the following supplements to help stabilize blood sugar:

- Chromium (200 micrograms per day)
- Alpha-lipoic acid (500 milligrams per day in divided doses)
- Vanadyl sulfate (5 milligrams per day)
- Zinc (5 to 15 milligrams per day)

Since alpha-lipoic acid can cause significant drops in blood sugar, start with small doses and work up. He can begin with 100 milligrams twice daily and work up to 500 milligrams with each meal.

He should eat eggs, garlic, onions, broccoli, asparagus, peppers, and Brussels sprouts, because these foods support the liver's detoxification processes. He can take the garlic as whole cloves, powder, or odorless garlic capsules.

Avoid iron-containing vitamins. Iron deficiency is very rare in men, and most of us get too much of it in our foods. In excess it has been shown to increase the risk of heart disease.

CHELATION THERAPY

EDTA (ethylenediaminetetraacetic acid) is a synthetic amino acid that was first used in the 1940s as an antidote to lead poisoning. If it is infused slowly into the bloodstream, it effectively binds heavy metals and dramatically reduces the production of free radicals. EDTA infusion, better known as *chelation therapy*, can clear blockages from arteries over a series of treatments, but it is considered an alternative medical practice by the American Medical Association. It competes with the lucrative business of heart disease drugs and surgeries offered by mainstream medicine. I predict that intravenous chelation will become standard disease-preventive therapy in the next few decades. If you are interested in finding out more about chelation, check the Resources section in the back of the book.

SUBSTANCES AND FACTORS THAT CONSTRICT BLOOD VESSELS

Like the plumbing in a house, the arterial system needs adequate pressure forces behind it to push fluids where they're needed. An intricate system of checks and balances exists to maintain arterial pressure so that your tissues receive an adequate blood supply. Blood pressure varies with activity level, and can double when we exercise. This dynamic equilibrium is accomplished by a marvelous interplay of the nervous and endocrine systems, incorporating the muscular blood vessel walls, the kidneys, the adrenal glands, and the sense organs.

High blood pressure, or hypertension, means that the pressure of blood within the arteries is above normal levels at rest. If the pressure rises, either the vessels are getting narrower or more fluid is passing through them than they're designed to hold. Both situations typically coexist. If efficiency of the systems that maintain fluid balance is decreased, salt and water retention is increased. The kidneys may not work as well as they once did, and so the excretion of water from the body may not happen fast enough.

The greatest damage due to hypertension is caused by the chronic constriction of blood vessel walls. Pressure mounts against the walls, raises the stress of flowing blood, and makes flow more turbulent. Any plaques that happen to jut out into the path of pressurized blood can easily be torn or burst, creating artery-clogging clots. The delicate capillaries are also susceptible to damage from high blood pressure.

If too much oxidized cholesterol or too much cortisol (stress hormones) is present, the body's artery-relaxing signals are blocked, and its blood vessels will remain clamped down.

A deficiency of the essential mineral magnesium also has the effect of blocking the body's natural blood-vessel-relaxation response. In a USDA study of 37,785 people, only 25 percent were taking in the recommended daily allowance of magnesium. Magnesium helps relax blood vessels and prevent arterial spasms and spasms of the heart muscle, but our soil and water stores are depleted of magnesium, and it isn't found in processed foods.

Calcium is also necessary for healthy blood vessels. Along with magnesium, the two minerals perform a constant balancing act throughout the body. Calcium constricts the muscular walls of the blood vessels; that's why calcium channel blocker drugs like nifedipine, verapamil, and diltiazem work to lower blood pressure.

Here's how calcium works. Imagine you're zooming along the highway one afternoon when someone starts tailgating you, even though you're obviously blocked from switching lanes to get out of his way. As your temper rises, calcium is released into your bloodstream, raises your blood pressure, and brings more blood to your brain and muscles so that you can function at a higher level of energy. Cortisol release also elevates blood pressure, and you are primed for fight-or-flight action. Magnesium is also released during stressful times to balance the effect of calcium, help you slow down, and keep your cool. If you don't get enough magnesium, the constrictive effect of calcium takes over and your blood pressure stays elevated. Eventually your body's blood pressure "thermostat" is reset to the higher numbers, and you're officially hypertensive.

THE ESSENTIAL FATTY ACIDS

There are two major classes of essential fatty acids necessary for good health: the omega-3s and the omega-6s, oils that we obtain through the foods we eat.

Omega-3 fatty acids are found in fish oils, flaxseed oil, canola oil, soy, walnuts, leafy greens and many other vegetables, sea vegetables, and pumpkin seeds. Omega-3s are changed in our bodies to *eicosapentaenoic acid* (EPA) and *docosahexaenoic acid* (DHA).

Omega-6 fatty acids are found in vegetable oils, leafy greens, most nuts and seeds, grains, and meats, as well as in the oils of borage, evening primrose, gooseberries, and black currants. Omega-6s are changed to *gamma-linoleic acid* (GLA) in our bodies.

EPA, DHA, and GLA are all involved in the production of specialized hormones called *eicosanoids*. There are several eicosanoids; some have a constricting effect on blood vessel walls and others have a dilating effect. An imbalance of omega-6 fatty acids in the diet means a preponderance of the artery-tightening eicosanoids. To make a long story short, most Americans get lots of omega-6s and not enough omega-3s, and their blood vessels are tensing up as a result. This is why it's so important to eat fish a few times a week, as well as plenty of fresh vegetables.

RX FOR BLOOD VESSEL CONSTRICTION

Stress management is key to blood vessel relaxation. Regular meditation, moderate exercise, or taking up a pleasant hobby are excellent stress-management techniques.

Magnesium supplementation is essential for anyone with high blood pressure. The drugs prescribed for hypertension further deplete already depleted magnesium levels, so *especially* if using prescription hypertension medication, take at least 400 milligrams of magnesium daily.

The amino acid arginine has the effect of improving cardiac function, lowering blood cholesterol, and increasing insulin sensitivity. It's a precursor to the body's blood vessel opener, nitric oxide. Your man should take 500 milligrams twice daily between meals.

Vitamin C supplementation loosens artery walls. He can take 1,000 milligrams at breakfast, lunch, and dinner. If diarrhea occurs, have him use a buffered form or reduce the dose by a few hundred milligrams.

He should consume fresh or fresh-frozen cold-water fish and other omega-3-rich foods such as pumpkin seeds. Minimize his exposure to oxidized fats, which means all unsaturated oils.

SUBSTANCES AND FACTORS THAT CAUSE THICKER BLOOD

Fibrinogen, oxidized cholesterol, "bad" eicosanoids, increased stickiness of platelets, and magnesium deficiency all contribute to the thickening of blood. It's like what happens to the oil in your car when it needs to be changed—it becomes sludgy and thick and likely to gum up the works.

Fibrinogen and platelets each play an essential role in the clotting of blood when you have a cut, but in the imbalanced state of the average Western male's bloodstream, there's too much fibrinogen and the platelets are too sticky. Chronic levels of high stress, smoking, and being overweight all contribute to excessive fibrinogen.

Deficiencies of magnesium and vitamin C are possible culprits in pushing *platelet aggregation* (collection of platelets around injuries) beyond what's needed. *Thromboxanes,* clotting elements needed to stop bleeding, are created in excess if there are too many omega-6 oils and too few omega-3 oils in the diet. Magnesium deficiency is also a suspected cause of blood clots.

Rx FOR THICK BLOOD

Garlic inhibits platelet aggregation and breaks down globs of fibrin. One clove of raw garlic per day will protect him from a long list of health problems. It should be taken with food, as it can cause stomach upset. If he opts for supplemental, odorless garlic, he should take 5,000 milligrams of allicin (garlic's active ingredient) per day. (The label should say how much allicin is in each dose.)

Vitamin C lowers fibrinogen levels, and vitamin E is a natural blood thinner.

Fish oils lower levels of thromboxane in the bloodstream. It's best to get them from eating fish, but supplemental fish oils also work. Look for the refrigerated kind or one that has been preserved to prevent it from becoming rancid. Follow the dosage directions on the container. Never take rancid fish oil.

HORMONE BALANCE AND BLOOD VESSEL HEALTH

Many hormones play pivotal roles in maintaining the health of the circulatory system. Men with higher testosterone and DHEA levels suffer fewer heart attacks. With testosterone replacement, "good" HDL cholesterol (which grabs excess blood cholesterol and takes it to the liver to be metabolized so that it doesn't end up stuck to artery walls) rises while "bad" LDL cholesterol drops.

Thyroid hormone, in adequate supply, dilates coronary arteries and increases the pumping strength of the heart. Thyroid hormone replacement improves the prognosis for heart patients with low thyroid hormone levels.

Growth hormone replacement enhances the sensitivity of the cells' insulin receptors, which means improved glucose uptake and lower blood insulin levels. Increases in HDL and decreases in body fat with HGH replacement mean decreased risk of artery disease.

BLOOD VESSEL SUPERNUTRIENTS

A few nutrients come as close as any substances can to being "magic bullets" in the treatment of artery disease. These natural therapies are beginning to be recognized and used by more mainstream doctors, because there's no denying that they work.

Coenzyme Q10
This coenzyme is an amazing, heart-supporting nutrient. It is part of the mitochondria of every heart cell and is responsible for energizing the network of smooth-muscle cells so that the heart beats strongly and regularly. CoQ10 levels fall in many diseases. People who have had heart attacks or who are in heart failure have incredibly low CoQ10 levels in their heart cells. Have your man take 30 to 200 milligrams per day of CoQ10 to energize the heart.

Soluble Fiber
Soluble fiber binds with cholesterol in the digestive tract and diminishes cholesterol absorption. Beans and oats are good sources of soluble fiber.

Gugulipid
This is a traditional ayurvedic medicine that effectively lowers blood cholesterol levels and consistently increases HDL cholesterol levels. It's derived from a tree resin and seems to do its work by increasing the number of binding sites for LDL in the liver. You can find it at your

health-food store. The recommended dose is 25 milligrams of guggul-sterones (the active ingredient) twice daily.

Carnitine

A nonessential amino acid, carnitine can be made in the body. It's responsible for transporting fatty acids into the mitochondria of cells (where energy is created from fuel) and for transporting wastes out. The heart muscle doesn't function as well when there's a shortage. It's deficient in those with heart disease, heart failure, and high blood fats. In one study of people with heart failure, carnitine relieved many of their symptoms, including swollen ankles, shortness of breath, and heartbeat irregularities. Your man can take 100 to 150 milligrams per day.

Lysine and Proline

These amino acids protect against deposits on blood vessel walls. Have him take 300 to 500 milligrams of lysine and proline three times a day.

12

Resisting the Diseases and Debilities of Aging

When we're born, we're a tiny package of rapidly dividing cells, our tissues expanding, lengthening, and finally reaching adult proportions. Although our growth phase begins to plateau in late adolescence, growth continues throughout our middle twenties. We can heap seemingly endless abuses on our bodies during this time, and in all but the most extreme cases, we can bounce right back to health.

Beneath the youthful exterior, however, changes in our bodies are beginning that may eventually cause our demise. Buildup of "gunk" inside coronary arteries starts before the tender age of five. Single cancerous cells can spring up during youth, lie dormant, or grow at a snail's pace for decades, until something triggers them to multiply out of control. Nutrient deficiencies and toxins wage microscopic wars against healthy cells. In our teens and twenties, our bodies can do whatever cleanup work is needed to stay ahead of these changes, and no outward symptoms of damage are evident. Somewhere in the third or fourth decade, though, the body can no longer keep up the damage control the way it once did.

At any age, the human body is able to continually remodel and replace its tissues; it is equipped with systems designed to maintain good, healthy tissues and dispose of any that are harmful or just taking up space. It's a dynamic equilibrium.

Just about everyone over thirty has a story to tell about the day they realized they were getting older, the day they got the message from their bodies loud and clear: "I just bent over to pick up a bag of groceries, and . . . wham! my back went out," or, "I used to be able to just go and go, nonstop energy, and suddenly I'm getting a sinus infection every time I have a big project due at work," and so on. The chorus to this plaintive song usually includes some variation of the phrase, "I'm getting old."

Aging is inevitable, especially for those who are fortunate enough to live for seven, eight, or nine decades. However, that downhill slope doesn't have to be steep. That's what this book is dedicated to: showing workable ways to shore up the decline, creating a gentle slope rather than a frightening roller-coaster ride. Hormone balance, minimizing stress, and getting the right nutrients are the tools to use for this roller-coaster renovation. Sure, we'll all have stiffer joints, catch colds easier, heal more slowly, and have less energy than we did when we were young. Our arteries will become less flexible and our organs will shrink over the years. These changes are simple facts of life at this point in human evolution. We're not perpetual-motion machines.

We've grown accustomed to the notion of debilitating illnesses as part and parcel of the aging process. However, there are a lot of disease processes that we can take steps to slow down or avoid as we age. With the right nutrition, supplements, and balance of hormones, men can dodge the diseases that cramp their styles as they age, or at least put off being affected by them for a few decades. Although it takes some work, and there are no guarantees, it is about playing the odds. Any man can improve his chances of enjoying the second half of his life thoroughly and in good health by taking specific steps now.

   This chapter will focus on causes, effects, and solutions for arthritis, aches and pains, colon cancer, osteoporosis, loss of vision, declining brain function, shrinking of the kidneys (and the resulting decrease in the ability to excrete toxins and maintain water and mineral balance), and sleep apnea (cessation of breathing for short intervals during sleep). All of these conditions, characteristic of the aging male, have specific causes and can be managed or corrected.

ARTHRITIS, ACHES AND PAINS, STIFFNESS, AND LOW BACK PAIN

Osteoarthritis is a common complaint among people over fifty-five. This type of arthritis is the result of a lifetime of wear and tear on joint tissues. Cartilage, which provides soft cushions between bones in the joints, is worn down, bringing bone rubbing against bone. Inflammation causes painful swelling in the joints and limited range of motion. Flareups of this degenerative disease can lead to permanent joint damage.

   Rheumatoid arthritis (RA) may feel a lot like osteoarthritis, but its origins are quite different. This is an *autoimmune* disease in which the immune system begins to destroy healthy tissues. Since several joints can be affected at once, extreme pain and decreased quality of life can result. Diets full of additives and food allergies have been implicated as causes of RA.

   RA affects people of all ages. The supplement, hormone, and diet advice that follow will work for relief of osteoarthritis and RA symptoms.

   Aches, pains, stiffness, and low back problems that plague so many are generally caused by overexercise or lack of exercise. In many cases, it's a little bit of both. Sitting still in a chair for hours at a time causes changes in the length and strength of muscles and tendons. Getting out of the chair and going for a run on a concrete sidewalk, without preparing the body for the stress, can result in injury. Microtears in the muscles or tendons and irritated joint capsules lead to inflammation and pain. Out-of-shape muscles can go into spasms that entrap nerves and cause pain, tingling, or numbness.

Regular exercise and stretching are the best ways to prevent aches and pains. The "weekend warrior" who is sedentary for days between short spurts of activity is the one most likely to get hurt. If your partner is the kind of person who constantly overdoes it, have him stop and evaluate his approach.

Do you know a man who can no longer spend the entire day playing touch football because he awakens the next morning so sore he can barely move? This is a natural transition, and it isn't necessarily one to be regarded with dread. It helps to think of it as an opportunity to gain in skill and finesse what is lacking in raw power. You might suggest that he cultivate a new efficiency of movement in his chosen activities and look out for his own safety. Look at the great dancer Mikhail Baryshnikov, who stunned audiences with his explosive power and speed in his youth. Now in his fifties, he is exploring new ways of dancing that are less acrobatic and more mature, refined, and centered.

Low back pain has reached epidemic proportions in the United States because of our sedentary lifestyle. To conquer low back pain, exercise, drop excess pounds, and try the stretches described in chapter 6. One shouldn't stay seated for too long at one time: Get up and move around every half-hour. Gentle backbends are good: Stand up straight with the heels of the hands planted on the back of the hips, roll the shoulders back, and lift the chest toward the ceiling. The face should turn up toward the ceiling, but the head shouldn't drop all the way back or the neck can be injured.

Those who are already dealing with painful arthritis are probably using anti-inflammatory medications on a regular basis. Nonsteroidal anti-inflammatory drugs (NSAIDs) like aspirin, ibuprofen and acetaminophen; steroids like prednisone; and injections of cortisone (for severe cases) are standard therapy for osteoarthritis. Although these medications are effective pain relievers, they can actually cause harm.

NSAIDs slow down the healing of cartilage and cause microtears in the lining of the small intestines, which can result in a leaky gut and all its attendant problems. High doses of powerful steroid drugs like prednisone quickly cause bone loss, weight gain, and a host of other side effects. Here are some other suggestions to alleviate arthritis pain and swelling:

- Try eliminating nightshade vegetables (tomatoes; potatoes; green, red, and other peppers; eggplant; and tobacco). It will take at least six weeks to see whether this helps.
- Use anti-inflammatory supplements like fish oil (omega-3 fats) and borage oil (omega-6 fats). Follow the dosage directions on the container.
- Hawthorn berry and bilberry contain powerful antioxidants that help minimize free radical damage in the joints. Take 200 to 400 milligrams per day of one of these bioflavonoids.
- Vitamin C is an essential component of *collagen,* out of which cartilage and all other connective tissue is made. Be sure to get adequate vitamin C, at least 2,000 milligrams and up to 10,000 milligrams (10 grams) daily.
- *Glucosamine sulfate* is a molecule necessary for the construction of *proteoglycans,* the raw material from which cartilage is made. Supplementation of 500 milligrams three times a day has brought about great improvement in arthritis patients, stimulating the manufacture of new, healthy cartilage.
- *Chondroitin sulfate* is another ingredient of cartilage, derived from glucosamine. It has shown promise as an arthritis fighter, especially when coupled with glucosamine sulfate.
- *Cetyl myristoleate* is a fatty acid found in a strain of mice known for its immunity from arthritis. It's being tested as a potential arthritis therapy. The standard dose is 600 milligrams per day.
- Hot pepper ointments (available from a health-food store), massage, gentle exercise (especially water exercise), and acupuncture are alternatives for coping with arthritis pain. If NSAIDs are

essential, be sure to supplement with L-glutamine, an amino acid that helps heal a leaky gut. Try 1,000 milligrams per day in divided doses between meals. Also try pantothenic acid (vitamin B₅) to rebuild intestinal walls; take 250 milligrams twice a day.

Several studies have made a connection between rheumatoid arthritis and low levels of DHEA, androstenedione, cortisol, and testosterone. Testosterone replacement produces significant improvement in those with RA; it seems to work by preventing the breakdown of collagen, the basic building blocks of connective tissue. If this is in fact how it works, it should be effective in osteoarthritis as well. Animal studies are showing DHEA's promise as an arthritis fighter. Small (physiologic) doses of natural hydrocortisone (5 to 10 milligrams with meals) can decrease inflammation without the awful side effects seen with synthetic corticosteroids like prednisone. For details on this approach, read *The Safe Uses of Cortisone* by William McK. Jefferies, M.D.

COLON CANCER

Cancer of the colon is directly linked to the typical Western diet of white flour and carcinogens. Diets very low in fiber slow down the transit of wastes through the large intestines. Waste sits for long periods in the colon (the bottom section of the large intestine), and whatever toxic chemicals your body has tried to get rid of have plenty of extra time to be reabsorbed. The continual exposure of the colon wall to poisons results in cancerous cell changes. A body that is chronically malnourished can't fight this process, so cancer cells grow out of control.

A health-supporting diet is the most important preventive tool against colon cancer. If there have been problems with constipation in the past, it is amazing the difference a whole-foods diet will make.

Some people find themselves having a bowel movement after each meal. Extra psyllium powder mixed with plenty of juice or water can be used when constipated. Simply mix the powder in eight ounces of fluid and drink before going to bed or before breakfast.

Dietary moderation may be the most important cancer-preventive tool we have. Animals that are given less to eat have fewer cancers, and the cancers they do have progress much more slowly than in animals allowed to eat as much as they like. Our "all you can eat" mentality is causing us to age earlier and die younger than we should. The solution is to eat only as much as you need and keep indulgences to a minimum.

The evidence that antioxidant nutrients play a pivotal role in the prevention of all cancers is incontrovertible. Each day, be sure to supplement the diet with these nutrients. (See chapter 5, "Keeping Cells Young by Squelching Oxidation.") Nutrients found in brassica family vegetables (broccoli, cauliflower, cabbage, brussels sprouts), garlic, and onions enhance the liver's ability to neutralize toxins. If foreign chemicals are neutralized, they won't do harm once they reach the colon.

Periodic internal cleansing is a good idea for those who don't eat an ideal diet. The liver is the body's most important cleansing organ. It filters toxins from the bloodstream and neutralizes them. You can support the cleansing function of the liver by taking milk thistle extract, also called *silymarin,* three times a day. Water or juice fasts that last from one day to five days give the body's healing systems a chance to repair damage throughout the gastrointestinal tract. For details on the whys and wherefores of fasting, read Ralph Golan, M.D.'s book *Optimal Wellness* or Joseph Pizzorno, N.D.'s *Total Wellness.*

Avoid regular consumption of known dietary carcinogens such as those found in fried foods, smoked foods, and foods containing nitrates (processed meats such as bacon and bologna). Avoid xenobiotic chemicals such as pesticides in foods as well.

Men who maintain youthful androgen (male hormone) levels will improve their resistance to colon cancer.

HOW TO STOP DECLINING BRAIN FUNCTION AND SLOWING OF NERVE IMPULSES

The Type A personality abounds in our culture. Even though we know it isn't the healthiest way to live, many men take pride in pushing themselves right up to their limits every day. These are the ones who insist that they thrive on stress, that they need so much stimulation to feel complete. Stress that is fun can be healthy. On the other hand, new research has shown that chronic stress kills: it clogs arteries, wears down the immune system, and unbalances our hormones. Furthermore, growing evidence links chronic stress and the release of the hormone cortisol to the deterioration of our brains as we age.

In a study reported in the April 15, 1998 issue of *Science News,* the cortisol levels of eleven elderly men and women were measured over a five-year span. Those with the greatest rise in free cortisol levels had the most deterioration of the *hippocampus,* a part of the brain responsible for memory and spatial orientation. This probably makes sense when we think about how forgetful and spacey we get when we're under the gun for long periods. These subjects also performed poorly on tests of these abilities in comparison to those with low levels of cortisol. In other words, someone who is constantly stressed is much more likely to become a forgetful old man who can't find his way back from the men's room.

The most important thing we can do to prevent brain deterioration due to stress is to become aware of how we're creating stress in our lives and then find creative ways to manage it better. We must learn to control the body's response to situations that cause the release of cortisol. Meditation creates a deeply relaxed, focused state that can carry over into all aspects of daily existence. For instance, if you're cut off by another car on the way to work, take deep breaths and tell yourself something soothing rather than letting yourself fly off the handle. After a while the calm response will come naturally, and the bursts of cortisol normally released in tense moments will diminish.

Cortisol release creates a kind of "high" that we crave after we come "down." We may unconsciously seek stressful situations or create a drama-trauma situation in our lives just to get that cortisol high. Eventually such behavior will take its toll on the adrenal glands and we won't be able to create a spike in cortisol levels because there will be nothing left to give. Tired adrenal glands will also make it hard to get up in the morning, and can lead to chronic fatigue and extreme fatigue after exercise.

AVOID ALUMINUM

Aluminum is a prime suspect in causes of Alzheimer's disease. Aluminum-containing antacids, foods packaged in aluminum cans or foil, aluminum cookware, baking soda, and underarm deodorants bring more aluminum into our bodies than we can get rid of. Avoid these products whenever possible. There are some great natural alternatives to conventional deodorants—look in the health-food store.

AVOID EXCITOTOXINS

Avoid the flavor enhancer MSG (monosodium glutamate) and the artificial sweetener aspartame. These food additives are *excitotoxins,* meaning that they have a potent excitatory effect on brain cells. In fact, brain cells become so excited that they self-destruct. Read labels carefully to eliminate these excitotoxins from your diet. MSG is well disguised in most foods these days as hydrolyzed vegetable protein or some variation on that theme. The best bet is to avoid processed foods, because almost all of them contain MSG.

Before you buy another can of diet soda, remember, not one study (and hundreds have been done) has ever shown that those who consume aspartame-sweetened sodas instead of sugar-sweetened sodas ever lost weight.

VITAMINS AND HERBS

The supplement plan we've discussed should deliver most of the nutrients needed by the brain to function optimally. The B vitamins and the antioxidants are particularly important. B vitamins keep brain cell metabolism going, and brain cell membranes are highly vulnerable to oxidation by free radicals. The inability to absorb vitamin B_{12} as we age is a major cause of senility. In such cases, oral sublingual (under the tongue) doses of vitamin B_{12} of 2,000 micrograms per day can turn the problem around within a matter of weeks.

Ginkgo biloba (up to 320 milligrams per day) and Siberian ginseng (follow the directions on the bottle) are herbs that enhance brain function.

The hormones pregnenolone and DHEA are helpful for those trying to improve brain function. Refer to the chapters on hormone balance to brush up on appropriate doses and uses of these natural hormones.

Melatonin, when used as a sleep aid, enhances the rejuvenating effect of deep sleep on brain chemistry. No more than 3 milligrams a few times a week should be used by a man under the age of sixty.

SHRINKING KIDNEYS

Chinese medicine says that the kidneys are an important center of *chi,* or life force energy. Kidney health is a barometer of the health of the rest of the body. The kidneys are balancing organs; when they aren't functioning well, several systems are thrown out of equilibrium.

The kidneys play several roles, including the excretion of toxins in the urine, maintenance of blood pressure, regulation of the acidity of the blood and body fluids, balance of electrolytes like potassium, calcium, and phosphorus, and the manufacture of blood components and some adrenal hormones.

Just like any other organ, the kidneys tend to shrink and function less efficiently as we age. High blood pressure, water retention, loss of minerals from bones (to regulate off-kilter acid-base balance), electrolyte imbalances (leading to heart arrhythmias and hypertension), and decreased ability to excrete toxins can all be indicators of deteriorating kidney function.

Overuse of the NSAID drugs such as aspirin, ibuprofen, and acetaminophen can eventually lead to kidney damage. Control pain and inflammation naturally whenever possible (for details, read the book *Prescription Alternatives* by Earl Mindell and Virginia Hopkins). Drink plenty of water between meals to keep diluted toxins flushing out through the kidneys. You should also avoid exposure to heavy metals like lead and mercury, because the kidneys are a primary storage depot for excess heavy metals. Lead is found in many places, including house dust, water, and fuels. Mercury is in many of our mouths as tooth fillings, and is also found in high concentrations in fish that live in shallow water (such as albacore tuna and shellfish). The presence of heavy metals sparks increased oxidation and death of kidney cells. Intravenous and oral chelating agents (see pages 168–169) remove these metals from the body.

Dandelion root is a well-known kidney tonic in natural medicine. Try drinking dandelion tea or eating dandelion greens in your salad.

VISION

For concerns about vision or if there is an eye disease that you'd like to treat naturally, read my book *Save Your Sight,* in which you will find detailed instructions about how to preserve eyesight and prevent or reverse eye disease.

Vision will most likely change for the worse as a man approaches andropause. The focusing mechanism—a set of tiny muscles that pulls on the lens of the eye and changes its shape to focus on objects that are close—becomes less able to do its job because the lens becomes less flexible. That's why people in their forties and fifties find that they have to hold text at arm's length to read it. A pair of reading glasses usually solves the problem. Even if the man in your life does not yet have vision problems, you should know that the healthier he keeps his blood vessels, the healthier his eyes will be. Taking those antioxidants and following my Eight Step program will help the eyes stay healthy longer.

Cataracts, glaucoma, and macular degeneration are eye diseases that can be linked to poor nutrition and exposure to toxins over the years. Here's a brief rundown:

- Cataracts affect two-thirds of Americans over the age of seventy. The lenses of the eyes become thickened and opaque. Symptoms include glare from lights at night and alteration of color perception. Excessive exposure of the eyes to sunlight and deficient antioxidant vitamins are to blame for most cases, so wear a good pair of UV-blocking sunglasses, eat right, and take those antioxidants. Fortunately, cataract surgery is a very simple procedure that completely cures the problem. Don't hesitate to have surgery if your vision is significantly impaired by cataracts.
- *Glaucoma* is a disease of the optic nerve. Nerve cells die and vision is lost from the periphery inward, so that there is a progressive "tunnel vision" that usually leads to total blindness. This disease is the most common cause of blindness in the United States. Conventional medicine treats glaucoma with powerful drugs that lower the pressure of the viscous fluid that surrounds the optic nerve. This isn't always the cause of the problem, and it doesn't do much to halt the progress of the disease. Steroid drugs, impaired circulation to the optic nerve (which is likely in blood vessel disease), and optic nerve toxins like MSG, cigarette smoke, and aspartame are all linked to glaucoma.

- *Macular degeneration* involves a tiny portion of the retina, the part of the eye that translates light rays into nerve impulses that travel through the optic nerve to the brain. Up to fifteen million people over the age of fifty are affected by macular degeneration. Like so many other diseases of aging, its causes can be traced back to poor diet, stress, and lack of exercise. Blood rich in nutrients and oxygen can't get to the retina because the tiny blood vessels that bring it there deteriorate. There are two kinds of macular degeneration. The less severe *dry* form usually involves blurring and waving of the visual field (like looking through the door of a shower stall). The *wet* form, with leaking of blood from damaged vessels, evolves from the dry form. New vessels begin to grow over the retina, blocking out vision at the center of the visual field. Macular degeneration doesn't rob one of all vision, but central vision can be completely destroyed. It's like having a big black disk right at the center of focus, with fairly intact peripheral vision.

To minimize the risk of these common diseases, follow the Eight Steps, wear sunglasses, and keep your antioxidant levels high. Leafy green vegetables, colorful fruits like cherries and blueberries, and deepwater fish are especially nourishing for the eyes. Supplements containing the bioflavonoids *lutein* and *zeaxanthin* supply the retinas with the nutrients they need to build new cells.

OSTEOPOROSIS

Men start out with about 30 percent more bone than their female counterparts, and so have less osteoporosis (literally, "porous bone"). That doesn't mean that men are immune, however. One-third of hip fractures happen in men, and men are more likely to die as a result of these fractures than are women. The important thing to remember about bone loss is that it starts as soon as levels of testosterone and growth hormone decrease. It creeps along over the years, bone break-down happening a little faster than bone buildup, and suddenly, at seventy or seventy-five, a man may break his hip or fractured his ver-tebrae and find himself permanently debilitated.

Testosterone and growth hormone replacement are the best weapons against bone loss. Amazing results have been achieved with these hormones in both men and women, halting the attrition of bone and even stimulating new bone formation. Regular weight-bearing ex-ercise, especially resistance training, has the same effect.

Adding calcium to the diet is important, too—try to do so with a wide variety of foods, including broccoli, leafy green vegetables, tofu, tempeh, almonds, and organic dairy products. Dietary supplements in the forms of calcium citrate or gluconate, 600 to 800 milligrams per day, are indicated. Vitamin D is needed for the proper use of calcium, so be sure that it's contained in a multivitamin, and get some sunshine every day (vitamin D is manufactured from cholesterol in the skin when we go out in the sun).

Anyone who drinks a lot of soft drinks should stop for the sake of their bones. Most sodas contain phosphoric acid, large amounts of which cause calcium to be pulled from the bones to buffer the extra acidity. The same goes for a very high-protein diet: protein foods are acidifying, and the body takes minerals from the bones to buffer ex-cess acid.

SLEEP APNEA

Any man who is frequently awakened at night by an ornery significant other who elbows him and hisses, "You're snoring—turn over!" or who finds himself growing very sleepy during the day may be suffering from *upper airway resistance* or *sleep apnea*.

If one snores often and wakes frequently during sleep, the airway is probably closing and temporarily cutting off the flow of air to the lungs. Less severe cases are categorized as upper airway resistance, while those who actually stop breathing five or more times an hour for ten seconds or more have sleep apnea. This potentially serious interruption of breathing can starve the brain and body of oxygen, and makes health-restoring sleep difficult. When the body keeps trying to pull air through closed-off airways, it causes an alarm response that wakes us. Stress hormones flood through the body to quickly arouse us. Awakening this way several times an hour during the night will make it very hard to get through the day.

Obesity is a common underlying cause of sleep apnea. Excess weight on the neck can compress the airways during deep sleep, when the muscles surrounding them are more relaxed. Normal-weight sleep apnea sufferers may have structural abnormalities that predispose them to the problem. People with hypertension, heart rhythm irregularities, heart failure, or past strokes or heart attacks are more likely to suffer from sleep apnea.

If you think the man in your life might be having episodes of sleep apnea, and you share sleeping quarters with him, tell him when he has been snoring and notice whether he is gasping, choking, or snorting in his sleep. He may be able to take care of the problem simply by quitting alcohol and other sedatives, losing some weight (if he's heavy), or sleeping in a different position (propped up with pillows or on one side). The next step is to see a physician for a sleep study to see whether treatment is indicated. Unfortunately, sleep apnea is not a problem that can treated with specific nutrients or hormones. If the changes I've mentioned here don't solve the problem, there may be a structural problem that needs medical attention.

Your physician may suggest a machine designed to create positive pressure in the airways with a continuous inflow of air. It plugs into a wall outlet and air is pumped through a mask or nasal tubes during the night. Oral appliances can be worn during the night, or medications may be prescribed. In some cases surgery can be performed to open a specific part of the airway.

BOOSTING THE IMMUNE SYSTEM

A healthy immune system is one that can accurately identify and dispose of unwanted invaders such as bacteria and viruses. It also targets and eliminates cancer cells before they have a chance to multiply out of control. Natural approaches to healing often work by potentiating the immune system.

There's a great deal one can do to fortify the immune system. Its function is greatly influenced by diet, lifestyle, and hormone balance. Regular moderate exercise enhances immune activity, and undue stress suppresses it. Eating a lot of sugar is a surefire way to hamper the immune responses.

Following my Eight Steps will provide excellent support for a strong immune system. When you feel a bug coming on, try the following immune-boosting formula:

- *Vitamin C:* This vitamin has amazing energizing effects on the immune system. Take up to 10,000 milligrams per day in divided doses.
- *Vitamin A:* Take 25,000 IU per day for up to two weeks.
- *Echinacea:* An herb that works by priming the immune system. Take up to 2,000 milligrams per day in capsule form until symptoms are relieved, in four 500-milligram doses throughout the day.
- *Goldenseal:* Another potent herbal germ fighter with direct bacteria-killing and immune-stimulating activity. Take up to 2,000 milligrams per day along with the echinacea.

- *Garlic:* Garlic has a remarkable capacity to stimulate the immune system. It fights bacteria, viruses, fungi, and parasites. Optimally, we should eat plenty of garlic whether or not we're sick, but take 1,500 to 1,800 milligrams per day of odorless garlic capsules when coming down with something, or mince a clove of raw garlic into a fresh salad.
- *Citricidal:* This standardized grapefruit extract is a nontoxic antibacterial now used in soaps and household cleaners. It can be taken orally to combat fungal, bacterial, parasitic, and viral infections.

The importance of the *thymus gland,* which nestles beneath the breastbone and begins to shrink in our thirties or forties, has been highlighted by recent research. No one is certain why it practically disappears in most people by the time they are in their seventies and eighties. We are certain, however, that replacing thymic hormones can have a dramatic effect on immune function. You can buy a supplement of thymus extract, usually extracted from calves' thymus glands. This is a good strategy for those who have frequent respiratory tract infections, cancer, or severe food allergies.

COMBATING DEPRESSION AND "MIDLIFE CRISIS"

Depression can happen at any point in a man's life. Some people suffer from it chronically throughout each stage of their lives, never really escaping it. Others don't experience depression until they begin to grow older. Feelings of hopelessness, sadness, and dread can make it difficult to fulfill responsibilities at work and at home. Depressed people often turn to drink, drugs, food, or sex to ease the discomfort temporarily.

Foods high in protein enhance mood by boosting growth hormone secretion. Carbohydrates, especially in sweets and high-fat junk food, enhance the release of the neurotransmitter *serotonin*—one that dictates mood. Eating junk when you're depressed actually is a form of self-medication. Antidepressant drugs like Prozac and Zoloft are *selective serotonin reuptake inhibitors* (SSRIs), which elevate mood by keeping serotonin active for a longer time in the space between neurons *(synapses)* in the brain. Before you turn to prescription drugs, try a few more natural routes.

St. John's wort *(Hypericum perforatum)* is an antidepressant herb that has become mainstream recently, and for good reason. Clinical studies have shown this ages-old remedy can provide relief from depression in as little as two weeks. It works every bit as well as prescription drugs and has fewer side effects. This natural SSRI blocks the reabsorption of serotonin, allowing it to remain active for longer periods. It inhibits an enzyme called *monoamine oxidase* (MAO), which breaks down the neurotransmitter *norepinephrine.* Raising levels of available norepinephrine elevates mood. MAO also breaks down serotonin in the synapses, so inhibiting it will also raise serotonin levels. Have him try 500 to 900 milligrams per day of standardized St. John's wort, containing 1 to 2.7 milligrams total hypericin, for at least one month. This herb shouldn't be used when taking prescription antidepressants (especially MAO inhibitors), sedatives, tranquilizers, cold or allergy medicines, amphetamines, narcotics, or the amino acids tryptophan or tyrosine, and alcohol and smoked or pickled foods should be avoided.

If it works, it can be continued for up to six months. In the meantime, do whatever psychological or spiritual work necessary to ferret out the causes of the depression. Psychological counseling, coursework on spiritual matters, or bodywork (such as massage)—or a mixture of the three—may be necessary to balance mind and body. An excellent resource on the psychology and spirituality of male menopause is Jed Diamond's book *Male Menopause.*

Andropause is not the same thing as midlife crisis, but they can certainly overlap. Midlife crisis is an emotional and psychological upheaval that may or may not coincide with dips in hormone levels. It usually occurs between the ages of thirty-five and forty-five, with the hormonal changes characteristic of andropause occurring between forty-five and fifty-five in most men. A man in the throes of midlife crisis may be depressed, anxious, fearful, and obsessive all at once. He feels unhappy with his lot in life, with his work and his spouse. He doubts the choices he has made and begins to dwell on how he may never attain the pinnacles of success and fulfillment he always imagined were within his reach. He feels inadequate and begins to fear his own aging and death. To cope with these feelings he may turn to sexual fantasy, alcohol, drugs, infidelity, or other escapes.

Men have not been encouraged to sit with their feelings or to turn to others for help. The fear of inadequacy and emasculation drive him to keep his fears and emotions locked in, and he begins to push others away so that they don't see through his ruse. Marriages break up as spouses drift further and further apart, perhaps taking other partners in an attempt to find the support and openness they don't have with each other.

Don't allow the man in your life to fall into the trap of midlife crisis. Understand that these feelings are normal and allow them to happen without acting rashly. Rather than solving problems by throwing money, food, or sex at them, encourage him to look within himself to their source. Reaffirm his values and his value as a man and a human being. Joining a men's group may give him a secure forum to air out his midlife crisis "dirty laundry," and once he's taken a good look at it he'll be better able to talk to you about it and live with it.

Decreased testosterone levels mean greater chance of depression. You know from chapters 3 and 4 that DHEA and growth hormone are potent mood-enhancers. Hormone replacement should go a long way toward relieving the depression and anxiety that can come with male menopause.

IN CLOSING

Bette Davis once said, "Aging is not for sissies." As with any challenge we face in our lives, we have a choice, and that choice will dictate whether we become blocked in our personal growth. We can be cowed by adversity and rely on others to show us the way out. We can throw up our hands and give up on making our lives better, continuing the grind because it's the only thing that makes us feel secure. Or we can take some risks, take charge of our health, remain proactive and aware of the changes in our bodies, and do what we can to improve the function of our various organs and prevent the onset of serious disease. To take responsibility for our own psychological and physiological health is the best way to grow through the challenges of andropause and reach new pinnacles of understanding and self-acceptance.

13

Dietary Strategies for Staying Power

A diet for staying power is rich in colorful organic vegetables; lean, hormone-free meats; fish and dairy products; nuts and seeds; eggs; whole grains; fresh fruits; unprocessed olive oil; and a variety of herbs and spices. Remember the cardinal rule of the Eight Steps: If it's in a package, processed with preservatives and mystery flavorings, it's not going to be good for you.

YOU ARE WHAT YOU EAT

Steaming, broiling, blanching (cooking quickly in boiling water), or light stir frying in olive oil, canola oil, or butter will bring out the best in nutritious foods. Raw organic vegetables are especially rich in nutrients. Avoid deep-fat frying or cooking with unsaturated oils like corn oil or safflower oil to reduce the risk of transforming an innocuous food like a potato or a chicken breast into a free radical load the body must struggle with to handle.

Polyunsaturated fats, which contain important essential fatty acids, are necessary for good health, but they are best eaten as components of nutritious foods, the way nature made them. Eating whole grains, vegetables, fruit, fish, and raw or lightly roasted nuts and seeds ensures getting plenty of unsaturated fats, well preserved against rancidity. Any fat heated to very high temperatures undergoes transformations into substances your body doesn't recognize, and that can be carcinogenic. Corn oil and safflower oil (polyunsaturates) are more unstable, and therefore more subject to this transformation with heating or sitting on the shelf, than are butter or coconut oil (saturates).

IF YOU'RE GOING TO SPLURGE, DO IT RIGHT

Which is the healthiest option?

- A big slice of real Bavarian chocolate cake from the mom-and-pop bakery, made with butter, sugar, real dark chocolate, cream, whole eggs, and flour? *or*
- A reduced-fat version from the supermarket, in which egg whites are substituted for whole eggs, margarine or other vegetable oils replace butter, and artificial sweetener replaces part of the sugar?

If you chose number two, I can hardly blame you. After all, that's the "wisdom" promulgated by the nutritional establishment, which advocates cutting fat and cholesterol as a pathway to good health. However, by replacing these essential and, unfortunately, demonized nutrients with fake fats and sugars, food manufacturers are doing you much more harm than good.

Americans have been convinced that these hybrid "plastic" foods promote health; that by virtue of having no fat and no cholesterol, a pretzel is better than an egg. The truth, however, is that the egg contains high-quality protein and fat-soluble vitamins, while the pretzel has primarily "empty calories," salt, a few vitamins added in after all the nutritional value of wheat has been processed out, and probably a hefty dose of chemical preservatives. The bottom line on the cake question is that you're far better off having a slice of the real thing than several unsatisfying chunks of the "low-fat" version.

CHOLESTEROL IS NOT A NUTRITIONAL VILLAIN

Cholesterol is made in the liver and is vital for survival. We need it to make our adrenal and sex steroid hormones, and it's a component of the body's cells. It's an essential component of cell membranes and nerve cells: besides creating a selectively permeable membrane around each cell, cholesterol squelches free radicals there as well. Cholesterol is needed to make bile, a substance manufactured in the liver that is necessary for the digestion of fats, and is needed to make vitamin D.

The liver keeps about 2,000 milligrams of cholesterol circulating in our blood at all times. Intake of dietary cholesterol, found in meats, chicken, fish, shellfish, organ meats, eggs, and dairy foods, usually results in a compensatory dip in the body's cholesterol production. Cholesterol rises in response to eating high-cholesterol foods only when we really overdo it. By now, I think we're all well aware that it's not healthy to eat red meat three times a day, seven days a week. Again, the principle of moderation comes into play. If we eat moderate amounts of saturated fats, our cholesterol should be fine.

A man over fifty who has been told by his physician that his cholesterol is too high has probably been given a prescription for a cholesterol-lowering drug. However, a cause-and-effect relationship between risk of artery disease and the amount of LDL ("bad") cholesterol in the bloodstream has not been established with any level of certainty. Researchers are coming to the conclusion that high levels of LDL are an *effect* of artery disease, not a *cause* of it.

It is actually much more important that he try to control the ratio of HDL ("good") cholesterol to LDL, and pay attention to when and if the LDL is oxidized. See chapter 5, "Keeping Cells Young by Squelching Oxidation."

HDL rises when we exercise; eat garlic, soy, and deepwater fish; and drink a few glasses of wine a week. Preventing the oxidation of LDL requires reducing chronic stress; getting plenty of antioxidant vitamins; and steering clear of toxic air, water, and food. Sounds a lot like the Eight Steps to me!

Prescription drugs to lower blood cholesterol are quite effective at creating a low cholesterol reading, but they don't always prolong or improve the lives of those who take them. They have a long list of negative side effects, and don't address the underlying cause of the high cholesterol; they only treat the symptom. Once again, it's a case of the pharmaceutical companies jumping at the results of a few studies, seeing the potential of a new drug to market, and the drug being over-prescribed to people who could attain better results by simply changing their lifestyles.

SUGAR AND ARTIFICIAL SWEETENERS

Norman is a sugar junkie. He's not ashamed—he'll tell you all about his sugar habit. "It rules my life," he says, "but I can't help myself— I've got such a sweet tooth!" He starts his day with a gargantuan mug of coffee, sweetened with two tablespoons of sugar and a dollop of nondairy creamer, and those iced toaster pastries his wife buys for the kids. By mid-morning he's lightheaded and sleepy, so he goes for a Pepsi and whatever sweet treats are set out in the break room at the office—usually Danish pastries, boxed low-fat brownies, or cookies. Lunch is a ham sandwich on rye at the deli around the corner and another coffee, and when the midafternoon slump strikes he steps out for a latte and a candy bar to tide him over until the magic hour of 5 P.M.

Do you know a guy like Norman? Is the man in your life a guy like Norman? Having a sugar habit may not seem like such an enormous problem—it's better than eating a lot of meat and eggs and cheese, right? Wrong. Sugar is being implicated as a causal factor in a host of degenerative illnesses, including heart disease and diabetes. Living with a sugar addiction pretty much guarantees a person will be in poor health, malnourished, subject to mood swings, and generally only able to perform far below capacity. Better to kick that sugar habit today and have staying power tomorrow.

Glucose, the simplest form of sugar, is the body's main source of energy. This complex molecule is the end-product of the breakdown of carbohydrates, and can be made from fats or proteins by special mechanisms in the liver if carbohydrate intake is inadequate. Our bodies shut down without a steady supply of glucose. If sugar is so important to survival, you might wonder why it is painted to be a nutritional no-no. The answer lies in the amount of processing the sugar has undergone when you consume it.

Glucose is the simplest sugar, and all carbohydrate foods, from broccoli to bread to lollipops, eventually are broken down into glucose by a complex series of chemical reactions that take place within the digestive tract. It flows through the circulation to each and every cell, where it's then broken down by another series of chemical reactions into energy and water.

Complex carbohydrates are foods as nature made them. Beans, brown rice, fruits and vegetables, and whole grains require a lot of processing within the digestive tract before they become glucose. The nutrients and dietary fiber contained in these complex carbohydrates are released during the digestive process and all play important roles in balancing glucose metabolism in the body and maintaining the health of the body that took them in.

Refined sugars like table sugar (sucrose), high fructose corn syrup, and maltodextrin are the products of intensive processing of sugar cane and the naturally occurring sugar in corn. They are stripped of nutrients, supplying nothing more to our diets than empty calories.

Unrefined honey, molasses, sugar cane juice, and maple syrup have very little nutrient value, but are slightly preferable to more refined sugar and vastly preferable to artificial sweeteners.

Table sugar is rapidly absorbed into the bloodstream when consumed because it's already "predigested." The nutrients the body needs to process complex carbohydrates are found in the foods themselves; when simple carbohydrates are eaten instead, the body has to draw from its precious stores of nutrients to get the job done.

The rapid rise in blood sugar levels that occurs when we eat sweets or refined flour creates a stressful, emergency situation in the body, where the first priority is to get blood sugar back within a normal range. A surge of insulin from the pancreas comes to the rescue, and blood sugar drops as abruptly as it rose. Although sugar may feel like a pick-me-up at first, there is a pronounced dip in energy levels soon after it's digested, so we take more. That puts us on the sugar-addiction treadmill.

Some people try to battle their sugar problem or cut calories by replacing the sugar in their diets with artificial sweeteners. Artificial sweeteners like aspartame aren't any healthier than the sugar they're used to replace, and there is evidence that aspartame is toxic to the nervous system. It gives many people severe headaches and dry eyes. Studies have shown that substitution of aspartame for sugar is more than compensated for in caloric intake—implying that people end up consuming more calories overall when they use aspartame-sweetened products!

The best way for anyone to kick the sugar habit is to quit cold turkey. Start on a day that won't be stressful, perhaps during a weekend, and eat nothing made with processed sugar, white flour, or artificial sweeteners. Take it easy on the fruit, too, because it is also high in sugar.

Have some unsweetened yogurt or slow-cooked oats for breakfast—not the processed, sugared kinds! Add a few slices of a ripe peach, banana, or strawberries. At the midday meal, enjoy some vegetable soup with a big green salad, and try a broiled salmon filet with a touch of lemon butter, dill, and thyme for dinner. Wild rice and some of the more bitter leafy greens like collards or kale go well with fish. Drink a lot of water, and try sipping green or black tea instead of coffee. It won't be easy at first, and everything may taste bland. Don't yield to the temptation to salt the food. Wean yourself off sugar, and retrain your palate to appreciate the subtler tastes of healthy, whole foods the way nature made them. If you can stay away from junk food and white flour for three months, I guarantee you'll feel better and will have gotten over any residual cravings. You'll notice a difference in as little as a few days.

Since sugar can weaken blood vessels, and you know what happens to a man's sex life when he has saggy blood vessels, consider sugar to be detrimental to your sex life.

DIET FADS: SORTING THE FACTS FROM THE FICTION

These guidelines should serve as a springboard to a lifetime of healthy eating. Notice I haven't addressed the issue of *diet composition*—the formula for determining how much fat, how much carbohydrate, and how much protein to eat each day. Over the past few years there has been hot debate over the optimal diet composition. Some swear by a very-low-carbohydrate, very-high-protein and unlimited-fat regimen, while at the other extreme there are those who insist that very-low-fat and very-low-protein diets consisting mainly of complex carbohydrates are the best approach. Most try a variety of approaches, often with mixed success. A typical problem is rebound weight gain when and if a dieter returns to normal habits.

A high-protein, high-fat diet very low in carbohydrates is based on the hypothesis that out-of-control insulin secretion in response to too many carbohydrates is to blame for the epidemic of obesity in America. Eggs, cream, cheese, and meats with vegetables and salads are the acceptable foods in these types of diets.

How can a person expect to lose weight on such a regimen? The reasoning is as follows: If you suppress insulin production by limiting carbohydrates, the body shifts into a metabolic mode called *ketosis* in which fat is broken down and used for fuel. The lack of carbohydrates sets the body into starvation mode, breaking down stored fats and proteins to make the needed glucose to keep your body going.

There are plenty of studies that show a link between high insulin levels and heart disease, and for some people this diet does bring diabetes under control, reduce cholesterol levels, and aid weight loss.

Another high-protein diet advocates a more moderate 40/30/30 ratio of carbohydrate to protein to fat. This eating plan can produce weight loss without feelings of deprivation. It can also improve mood, concentration, and energy levels for some people. This diet also tends to work well for diabetics and others with sugar control problems.

On the other end of the spectrum are the low-fat, high-complex-carbohydrate, vegetarian regimens. Again, clinical studies have shown that a diet very low in fat and rich in complex carbohydrates, along with exercise and stress reduction, can quickly and dramatically improve the health of those with coronary artery disease. Researchers have shown that life-threatening heart vessel blockages can be reduced in some people with these interventions. For many people who adhere to these types of diets, body weight, blood fats, fasting blood sugars, and insulin levels drop consistently.

Confusing, isn't it? I'd like to clear things up and in the process show how to figure out the best way to keep body weight and insulin levels under control.

It is absolutely true that Americans continue to get fatter despite the widespread consumption of foods low in fat and artificially sweetened. The number of people with health problems related to out-of-control insulin levels continues to rise unabated, and the mainstream medical solutions usually include powerful drugs that cause more illness than they relieve. Treating a single symptom, such as high cholesterol or high blood sugars, with a single "magic bullet" drug tends to knock the body even further out of balance. It follows that using a diet specifically designed to affect one metabolic variable, such as high insulin or cholesterol levels—the "food as medicine" approach—may have a similar, yet more subtle effect. Again, the magic word is *moderation*.

No One Plan Works for Everyone

Where most popular "diet plans" go wrong is in their steadfast insistence that one must follow them to the letter. The assumption is that the same diet works the same way in all people's bodies. We may be members of the same species, but the biochemical variety that exists within that species is enormous. No one approach is the answer for everyone.

The best diet for each of us depends on the interaction between our particular set of genes and our environment. My advice is to start keeping a food journal over the next few weeks. Record what you eat, when you eat it, and how you feel before and after you eat. Include notes about your general health and well-being. If you notice that your diet is heavy on the refined carbos (bread, pastries, sweets, "low-fat" snacks), try a regimen that replaces those foods with vegetables, small servings of complex carbos like brown rice, and protein foods like meat, eggs, soy, and fish. You'll probably lose a few pounds and feel a lot better.

If either of you is addicted to fatty foods and is displeased with the way you feel and look, it won't help to try to completely deprive yourself of fat. The first thing you need to do is cut out the hydrogenated oils and margarines. That will mean eliminating nearly all processed foods, especially chips, cookies, and other baked goods.

When you do eat fat, use small amounts of butter and olive oil in your cooking, and small amounts of meat, nuts, seeds, and dairy products. Emphasize generous helpings of vegetables, some fruit, and whole grains.

If either of you suffers from chronic sinus or respiratory ailments, eliminate dairy products (milk, cheese, ice cream, yogurt) for a couple of months and see if the problem clears up. Dairy products can increase mucus production and cause congestion.

Chronic gastrointestinal distress with bloating, constipation, and diarrhea may have been diagnosed as "irritable bowel syndrome" by a physician. However, that may be incorrect. What may be irritating the bowel is either an intolerance to milk protein (lactose intolerance) or the protein gluten found in many grains, especially in wheat (gluten intolerance). Try eliminating each food from your diet and reintroducing them after six weeks. An intense reaction indicates an allergy or intolerance; substitute other foods for those from that point on.

Food allergies don't necessarily make a person sneeze or break into hives. However, they tend to have subtle and pervasive effects throughout the body and cause fatigue and general malaise. Food allergies and intolerances are most often triggered by the foods we eat every day and can't imagine going without. We tend to be addicted to the foods we're allergic to. Some alternative medicine specialists theorize that the allergy/addiction process is created when the body releases adrenaline in response to the allergen, creating a temporary boost in energy.

Make a list of the foods that each of you feel you absolutely must have every day—for most people, wheat or dairy products are at the top of the list. Foods containing soy, shellfish, eggs, and peanuts are other common food allergens. Systematically eliminate each food on your list for one or two weeks and see how you feel.

"GOOD" FOODS, "BAD" FOODS

EGGS

Eggs have been much maligned over the past decade. Each egg, with its 217 milligrams of cholesterol, has been wrongly characterized as an artery-clogging decadence. Dietary recommendations have been to limit egg consumption to no more than three or four a week, and anyone who consumes the typical meat-rich, highly processed American diet *should* follow those guidelines. Someone who eats a healthful, whole foods-based diet, however, can enjoy eggs more often and suffer no ill effects. Remember to buy organic, cage-free eggs to avoid eating the hormones and chemicals given to caged, laying hens in factory farms.

Eggs can be an important source of essential amino acids and fatty acids for vegetarians. An egg or two every couple of days can help boost their protein intake if they feel the need to supplement the beans, rice, whole grains, and corn that satisfy a vegetarian's daily protein requirements.

MILK AND DAIRY PRODUCTS

Milk products are advertised as a necessary source of dietary calcium. It's true that milk contains calcium that your body can use, but let's consider the vehicle. Cow's milk is food for calves, and it contains proteins the human body may not be equipped to digest properly. Some people are unable to break down *lactose,* or milk sugar, because they don't make the necessary enzyme, *lactase.* In those who are lactose-intolerant, the milk sugar molecules pass through the digestive tract without being broken down and are broken down in the large intestines by the bacteria that reside there. This results in the production of large amounts of gas, painful intestinal spasms, and (often) diarrhea. Lactose intolerance is most common in people of African-American or Asian descent and least common in people of Scandinavian descent.

Some lactose-intolerant people can eat some dairy products such as hard cheeses and butter, which are very low in lactose. Digestive aids like Lactaid can supply the lactase needed to digest other dairy.

Milk undergoes a great deal of processing during its journey from cow's teat to your table. Some (whole or 2 percent milk) or all (skim milk) fat is removed, and the remainder is *homogenized* to evenly distribute fat molecules through the liquid. There is some evidence that homogenization of milk renders it harmful to the blood vessels. Homogenization causes an enzyme contained in the milk to pass into the bloodstream of the person who consumes it. This enzyme damages the wall of the arteries, and this sort of damage is the first step in the cascade of events that leads to the development of an arterial plaque.

Most milk is heated to high temperatures, or *pasteurized,* to kill bacteria. Unfortunately, pasteurization also kills enzymes that are an important part of milk, and which aid in its digestion. Pasteurized milk is dead food. Small servings of pasteurized milk, yogurt, or cheese every so often are fine, but daily consumption of highly processed dairy is a bad idea. Those who are allergic to dairy products can try eating raw milk and cheese from a reputable local dairy.

BUTTER AND OTHER SATURATED FATS

Butter has also been labeled a dietary menace by the so-called nutrition experts. Saturated fats, in general, have been on the long list of undesirable foods since a relationship was reportedly found between consumption of these fats and risk of heart disease. Polyunsaturated fats were suddenly the "heart-healthy" way to go. As is often the case in that netherworld between science and advertising, insufficient evidence of a cause–effect relationship was transformed into booming sales of so-called "heart-healthy" processed foods. Now the pendulum is swinging back in the other direction, and it's turning out that it's best to use *small amounts* of the more stable saturated versions (butter) than the overprocessed hydrogenated oils (margarines and vegetable shortenings) or the unsaturated oils, which are almost always rancid.

If polyunsaturated oils aren't stabilized with the hydrogenation process, they easily become rancid: As fat molecules become oxidized, they start the cascade of free radical formation in the body when we eat the oil. When polyunsaturates are heated even a little in cooking, a free radical load is created that may not be worth those french fries, chips, or fried chicken.

It is safe to use a small amount of butter on food, but going beyond the moderation zone is asking for trouble. Olive oil is the gold standard for cooking. In study after study, the health benefits of olive oil far exceed those of any other cooking oil.

SOY FOODS

Soy is being hailed as a superfood these days, but don't get carried away with it. Limit intake of fermented soy foods to two or three times a week. Unfermented soy contains substances that block protein digestion, glucose uptake in the brain, and mineral absorption, and interfere with thyroid function. Soy milk and untreated soy proteins are some of the worst culprits when it comes to these toxic effects. The traditional Asian methods of preparing soy—tofu, tempeh, and miso—appear to be the most healthful.

THE IMPORTANCE OF CALORIC INTAKE

All the sensible diets share a few common threads: few or no processed foods, generally low in total calories, very little or no sugar, plenty of vegetables, and ingredients that are fresh, organic, and untainted. This is the happy middle ground.

One very exciting area of research right now has shown that simple caloric restriction—eating less food—dramatically increases the longevity of test animals. Not only do these animals live longer lives, they suffer from far fewer illnesses than do control animals allowed to eat as much as they like.

The mechanism for the preservation of youth and life extension appears to be the reduction in the amount of wear-and-tear on the body. Overconsumption of food places a burden on the body. Excess calories and nutrients have to be broken down and either stored or excreted. More free radicals are produced.

In contrast, when less food is consumed, the body learns to use energy more efficiently. This doesn't mean to starve yourself, but to try eating more consciously and deliberately. Chew each bite thoroughly and experience the flavors and textures. Stop when you're satiated rather than stuffed. Enjoy small portions of really delicious foods rather than massive portions of bland foods.

14

Dr. Marc's Prescription for Staying Power

Here's a quick reference for your partner to use in this anti-aging program. It includes summaries of supplement, nutrition, and hormone recommendations from each chapter. (See Table 14.1.)

Table 14.1 Men Need Hormone Balance, Too

Hormone	Indications	Dosage
Transdermal crystalline testosterone as gel or patch applied daily*	All symptoms of male menopause, arthritis	Enough to raise blood levels of free testosterone to 900–1,200 mcg/ml and salivary levels to 30–40 mcg/ml
Micronized DHEA	Low energy, depression, arthritis; have a salivary DHEA test to see if you're deficient	10–25 mg/day
Pregnenolone	Forgetfulness, difficulty thinking straight	100 mg/day between meals
Androstenedione†	General symptoms of andropause; difficulty building muscle with resistance training	50–100 mg two to five times weekly
Natural progesterone	Hair loss, overexposure to xeno-estrogens, prostate problems	5–10 mg daily as a cream used locally
Natural hydrocortisone*	Chronic fatigue, autoimmune disease, inflammatory conditions such as arthritis; have a salivary cortisol test to see if you are low	5–20 mg/day divided into 5-mg doses with food

* Available by prescription only.
† Available over the counter, but use should be supervised by a physician.

THE ANTI-AGING HORMONES

GROWTH HORMONE

Human growth hormone: physiologic doses injected twice a day,
under the close supervision of an anti-aging physician

Natural growth hormone boosters: exercise, weight loss, quality
sleep, periodic fasts one to three days long, foods rich in
protein

Amino acids that raise growth hormone levels: arginine and lysine,
1,200 to 1,500 milligrams each, increasing to 3,000 milligrams
each over time; ornithine, glutamine, and glycine can also be
added, starting with 500 milligrams each and increasing to
1,000 milligrams or more

Niacin: the no-flush variety, 200 to 500 milligrams, starting with
50 milligrams

Prescription drugs that increase growth hormone secretion:
L-dopa, hydergine, phenytoin, clonidine

INSULIN

Chromium picolinate: 100 to 200 micrograms per day

Vanadyl sulfate: 5 to 10 milligrams per day

Alpha-lipoic acid: 500 milligrams per day in divided doses
(may cause dip in blood sugar)

Vitamin C: 1,000 to 2,000 milligrams

Quercetin: 500 to 1,000 milligrams per day

Omega-3 fatty acids in deepwater fish

Garlic: raw or cooked cloves or odorless capsules, equivalent of
5,000 milligrams allicin per day

Zinc: 10 to 15 milligrams per day

MELATONIN

Improves sleep habits: don't use bed for reading, working, or
watching TV; keep sleep-wake cycles regular; don't drink caffeinated beverages or eat chocolate after 3 P.M.; don't exercise
within three hours of bedtime, but do exercise every day
if possible

High–complex carbohydrate snack to enhance secretion of
tryptophan

Calcium/magnesium tablet an hour before bed, 400 and
300 milligrams, respectively

Valerian: follow dosage instructions on container; take as a tincture
or capsule of dried herb an hour before bed

Melatonin: 1 to 3 milligrams by tablet or sublingually one hour to
a half-hour before bed; no more than three times a week

DIETARY STRATEGIES FOR STAYING POWER

MULTIVITAMIN GUIDELINES

Always choose an iron-free multivitamin, unless you have been diagnosed with anemia or iron deficiency. Doses below are per day.

Beta carotene/carotenoids: 10,000 to 15,000 IU
Vitamin A: 5,000 to 10,000 IU
The B vitamins:
    Thiamine (B_1): 25 to 50 milligrams
    Riboflavin (B_2): 25 to 100 milligrams
    Niacin (B_3): 50 to 100 milligrams
    Pantothenic acid (B_5): 50 to 100 milligrams
    Pyridoxine (B_6): 50 to 100 milligrams
    Vitamin B_{12}: 1,000 to 2,000 micrograms
    Biotin: 100 to 300 micrograms

Choline: 50 to 100 milligrams
Folic acid (folate or folacin): 400 to 800 micrograms
Inositol: 150 to 300 milligrams
Calcium: 300 to 500 milligrams
Vitamin D: 100 to 400 IU
Vitamin C: 2,000 to 10,000 milligrams
Vitamin E: 400 IU
Boron: 1 to 5 milligrams
Chromium: 200 to 400 micrograms
Copper: 1 to 5 milligrams
Magnesium: 300 to 500 milligrams
Manganese: 5 to 10 milligrams
Selenium: 50 to 200 micrograms
Vanadyl sulfate: 5 to 10 milligrams
Zinc: 10 to 30 milligrams

KEEPING CELLS YOUNG BY SQUELCHING OXIDATION

GLUTATHIONE BOOSTERS

Sulfur-containing foods (eggs, onions, garlic, asparagus)
Alpha-lipoic acid: 500 milligrams per day in divided doses
N-acetyl-cysteine: 500 milligrams two to three times a day
Milk thistle (silymarin): 120 milligrams three times a day as dried
    herb (in capsules) or tincture (two drops in water)
Coenzyme Q10: 30 to 200 milligrams per day
Melatonin: 1 to 3 milligrams a few times a week before bed

The Antioxidant Arsenal

Vitamin C: 1,000 to 2,000 milligrams per day in divided doses;
two to five times more when sick (use buffered forms like calcium or magnesium ascorbate if taking more than 2 grams
per day)

Vitamin E: 400 IU per day

Beta-carotene (provitamin A): 10,000 to 15,000 IU per day

Carotenoids (lycopene, lutein, zeaxanthin): in spinach, collards,
kale, and other leafy greens; have these foods at least twice
a week

Selenium: 200 milligrams per day

Anti-inflammatory Antioxidants

Quercetin: 500 to 1,000 milligrams per day

Omega-3 oils in fish

MAINTAINING MUSCLE FOR LIFE

Creatine phosphate: use a powdered form, starting with a loading
dose of 15 to 20 grams per day in four divided doses for one
week, then continuing with 3 to 5 grams per day

Branched-chain amino acids (leucine, isoleucine, valine): follow
the instructions on the container

Coenzyme Q10: 60 milligrams per day

Chromium: 100 to 200 micrograms per day

Ginseng: 1 to 2 grams per day of ginseng containing 4 percent to
7 percent ginsenosides

KEEPING UP IN THE BEDROOM

Yohimbine: as Yocon or Yohimbex by prescription; use only occasionally just before sex

Ginkgo biloba: 320 milligrams per day

Ginseng: 1 to 2 grams per day of ginseng containing 4 percent to 7 percent ginsenosides

Saw palmetto: 160 milligrams twice a day

Other herbs: ashwaghanda, wild oats *(Avena sativa), Urtica dioica,* damiana *(Turnera aphrodisiaca)*

PROTECTING HIS PROSTATE

Saw palmetto: 160 milligrams per day; formulas with this herb may include *Pygeum africanum* and nettle root

Beta sitosterol (extract of saw palmetto; use either whole herb or extract): 60 milligrams per day

Panax ginseng: 25 to 50 milligrams ginsenosides per day

Zinc picolinate: 15 to 30 milligrams per day for six months

Pumpkin seeds for zinc and omega-3 fatty acids

Vitamin B_6: 50 milligrams per day

KEEPING HIS HAIR ON HIS HEAD

Fresh fish, kelp, dulse, nori, at least twice a week for iodine

Vitamins E, A, and C as recommended in diet and oxidation chapters

B complex

B_6: 50 milligrams per day

Mineral hair health formula containing silica, magnesium, calcium, selenium, potassium, and phosphorus

KEEPING HIS BLOOD VESSELS CLEAR AND STRONG

SUPPLEMENTS TO CLEAR OUT BLOOD VESSELS

Vitamin C: 3,000 milligrams per day in divided doses

Vitamin E: 400 IU per day

N-acetyl-cysteine: 500 milligrams two to three times a day

Quercetin: 125 to 250 milligrams three times a day

Bromelain: 125 to 250 milligrams three times a day

Ginkgo biloba: 320 milligrams per day

Mixed flavonoid supplement (quercetin, rutin, bilberry, grapeseed extract, green tea)

Folate: 50 micrograms per day

Vitamin B_6: 50 milligrams per day

Vitamin B_{12}: 800 micrograms sublingually or intranasally

SUPPLEMENTS FOR ADULT ONSET DIABETES

Chromium picolinate: 100 to 200 micrograms per day

Vanadyl sulfate: 5 to 10 milligrams per day

Alpha-lipoic acid: 500 milligrams per day in divided doses (may cause dip in blood sugar)

Vitamin C: 1,000 to 2,000 milligrams

Quercetin: 500 to 1,000 milligrams per day

Omega-3 fatty acids in deepwater fish or fish oils

Garlic: odorless capsules, equivalent of 5,000 milligrams allicin per day

Zinc: 10 to 15 milligrams per day

SUPPLEMENTS TO RELAX BLOOD VESSEL WALLS

Magnesium: 200 to 400 milligrams per day
Arginine: 500 milligrams twice a day
Deepwater fish, pumpkin seeds (for omega-3 fatty acids)

SUPPLEMENTS TO MAKE BLOOD FLOW MORE FREELY

Garlic: enough odorless capsules to total 5,000 milligrams allicin
Fish oil from deep-sea fish

BLOOD VESSEL SUPERNUTRIENTS

Coenzyme Q10: 30 to 200 milligrams per day
Soluble fiber from beans, grains, ground flaxseeds
Gugulipid: 25 milligrams guggulsterones three times a day
Proline and lysine: 300 to 500 milligrams of each three times
   a day
Carnitine: 100 to 150 milligrams per day

RESISTING THE DISEASES AND DEBILITIES OF AGING

ARTHRITIS

Eliminate nightshade vegetables (tomatoes, potatoes, green pep-
   pers, red peppers, eggplant, tobacco) for at least six weeks
Hawthorn berry or bilberry: 200 to 400 milligrams per day
Vitamin C: at least 500 milligrams per day
Glucosamine sulfate: 500 milligrams three times a day
Chondroitin sulfate: use with glucosamine
Hot pepper ointments, gentle exercise, acupuncture, bodywork
   for pain

To counter intestinal damage from NSAIDs: L-glutamine
(1,000 milligrams per day in divided doses), pantothenic acid
(vitamin B$_5$: 50 milligrams twice a day)
Testosterone replacement
DHEA replacement
Natural hydrocortisone: 2.5 to 5 milligrams four times a day

Colon Cancer

Plenty of dietary fiber; supplement with psyllium
Full antioxidant protection as described in chapter 5
Milk thistle and alpha-lipoic acid
Periodic internal cleansing and fasting
Avoid known dietary carcinogens: nitrates, fried or smoked foods
Melatonin: 1 to 3 milligrams no more than three nights a week

Memory Loss

Decrease stress and manage it better
Avoid aluminum-containing deodorants and antacids
Avoid MSG and aspartame
Ginkgo biloba: 320 milligrams per day
Siberian ginseng: 100 milligrams per day of extract containing
1 percent eleutherosides
CoQ10: 100 milligrams per day
Pregnenolone replacement
DHEA replacement
Melatonin: 1 to 3 milligrams no more than three times a week

PRESERVING VISION

Leafy greens: kale, collards, spinach
Deepwater fish
Supplement for eye health containing lutein and zeaxanthin

BOOSTING IMMUNITY

When you start to come down with something:

Vitamin C: 2,000 to 6,000 milligrams per day in divided doses
(use the buffered forms—calcium or magnesium ascorbate—if
higher doses upset your stomach, or reduce the dose)
Vitamin A: 15,000 to 25,000 milligrams per day of preformed vitamin A for up to two weeks
Echinacea: up to 2,000 milligrams per day in divided doses
Goldenseal: up to 2,000 milligrams per day in divided doses
Garlic: 1,500 to 1,800 milligrams per day of odorless capsules, and
use fresh or powdered garlic liberally on food
Thymic hormone replacement: follow the directions on the container; if you are very susceptible to infection, or have severe
food allergy or cancer, take this on an ongoing basis

OSTEOPOROSIS PREVENTION

Testosterone and growth hormone replacement
Calcium citrate/gluconate and magnesium: 600 milligrams per day
and 400 milligrams per day
Vitamin D: 100 to 400 IU daily, some exposure to sunlight
Avoid soft drinks

HEALING DEPRESSION AND MIDLIFE CRISIS

St. John's wort: 500 to 900 milligrams per day of extract containing 1 to 2.7 percent total hypericin for at least one month
Counseling, spiritual exploration and practices, bodywork, turning
to loved ones when needed

Resources

ANTI-AGING PHYSICIAN REFERRALS

The American Academy of Anti-Aging Medicine (A⁴M):
   (773) 528-4333

CHELATION

The American College for Advancement in Medicine
   P.O. Box 3427, Laguna Hills, CA 92654
   1-800-532-3688 (outside California)
   (714) 583-7666 (in California)

FLUORIDATION

Call (301) 874-2948 to subscribe to a quarterly newsletter, *The Fluoride Report,* devoted to the fluoridation debate.

LASER SURGERY

The American Society for Dermatologic Surgery: 1-800-441-2737, www.asds-net.org

The American Society of Plastic and Reconstructive Surgeons' Plastic Surgery Information Service: 1-800-635-0635

BriteSMILE, a network of dentists that practice laser tooth whitening: 1-800-272-7375, http://britesmile.com

RECOMMENDED READING

Walsh, Patrick C., and Janet Farrar. *The Prostate: A Guide for Men and the Women Who Love Them.* Baltimore: Johns Hopkins University Press, 1995.

Mindell, Earl, and Virginia Hopkins. *Prescription Alternatives.* Los Angeles: Keats Publishing, 1998.

Eades, Michael, and Mary Dan Eades. *Protein Power.* New York: Bantam Books, 1996.

References

CHAPTER 1:
IS MALE MENOPAUSE A MYTH?

de Lignieres, B. "Transdermal Dihydrotestosterone Treatment of 'Andropause'." *Annals of Medicine* 25(3): 235–41 (June 1993).

Green, James. *The Male Herbal: Health Care for Men and Boys.* Freedom, Calif.: The Crossing Press, 1991.

Vermeulen, A. "Environment, Human Reproduction, Menopause, and Andropause." *Environmental Health Perspectives* 101, Suppl 2: 91–100 (July 1993).

CHAPTER 2:
EIGHT STEPS TO STAYING POWER FOR LIFE

Golan, Ralph, M.D. *Optimal Wellness.* New York: Ballantine Books, 1995.

Hallwell, B. "Free Radicals, Antioxidants, and Human Disease: Curiosity, Cause, or Consequence?" *The Lancet* 344 (Sept. 10, 1994).

Khalsa, D. S. "Science, Spirituality and Longevity: Where the Evidence Stands." *Anti-Aging Medical Therapeutics.* Marina Del Rey, Calif.: Health Quest Publications, 1997, pp. 157–60.

Khalsa, Dharma Singh, and Cameron Stauth. *Brain Longevity.* New York: Warner Books, 1997.

Klatz, Ronald, M.D. *Grow Young with HGH.* New York: Harper Collins, 1997.

Mindell, Earl, and Virginia Hopkins. *Prescription Alternatives.* 2d ed. Los Angeles: Keats Publishing, 1999.

Smith, G. D., S. Frankel, and J. Yarnell. "Sex and Death: Are They Related? Findings from the Caerphilly Cohort Study." *British Medical Journal* 315: 1641–44 (Dec. 1997).

Steinman, David, and Michael Wisner. *Living Healthy in a Toxic World.* New York: The Berkeley Publishing Group, 1996.

Walker, Morton, M.D. *The Chelation Way.* Garden City, N.Y.: Avery Publishing Group, 1995.

CHAPTER 3:
MEN NEED HORMONE BALANCE, TOO

TESTOSTERONE
Arver, S., et al. "Improvement of Sexual Function in Testosterone Deficient Men Treated for 1 Year with a Permeation Enhanced Testosterone Transdermal System." *Journal of Urology* 155(5): 1604–8 (May 1996).

Bellido, T., et al. "Regulation of Interleukin-6, Osteoclastogenesis, and Bone Mass by Androgens. The Role of the Androgen Receptor." *Journal of Clinical Investigation* 95 (6): 2886–95 (June 1995).

Bhasin, S., et al. "Testosterone Replacement Increases Fat-Free Mass and Muscle Size in Hypogonadal Men." *Journal of Clinical Endocrinology and Metabolism* 82 (2): 407–13 (Feb. 1997).

Bhasin, S., et al. "The Effects of Supraphysiologic Doses of Testosterone on Muscle Size and Strength in Normal Men." *New England Journal of Medicine* 335(1): 1–7 (July 4, 1996).

Brodsky, I. G., P. Balagopal, and K. S. Nair. "Effects of Testosterone Replacement on Muscle Mass and Muscle Protein Synthesis in Hypogonadal Men—A Clinical Research Center Study." *Journal of Clinical Endocrinology and Metabolism* 81(10): 3469–75 (Oct. 1996).

Carruthers, M., M.D., F.R.C.Path., M.R.C.C.P. *Male Menopause: Restoring Vitality and Virility.* London: HarperCollins, 1996, p. 90.

Flood, J. F., J. E. Morley, and E. Roberts. "Memory-Enhancing Effects in Male Mice of Pregnenolone and Steroids Metabolically Derived from It." *Proceedings of the National Academy of Sciences of the United States of America* 89(5): 1567–71 (March 1, 1992).

Glueck, C. J., et al. "Endogenous Testosterone, Fibrinolysis, and Coronary Heart Disease Risk in Hyperlipidemic Men." *Journal of Laboratory and Clinical Medicine* 122 (4): 412–20 (Oct. 1993).

Guo, C. Y., T. H. Jones, and R. Eastell. "Treatment of Isolated Hypogonadotropic Hypogonadism Effect on Bone Mineral Density and Bone Turnover." *Journal of Clinical Endocrinology and Metabolism* 82 (2): 658–65 (Feb. 1997).

Haffner, S. M., et al. "Low Levels of Sex Hormone-Binding Globulin and Testosterone Are Associated with Smaller, Denser Low Density Lipoprotein in Normoglycemic Men." *Journal of Clinical Endocrinology and Metabolism* 81(10): 3697–701 (Oct. 1996).

Katznelson, L., et al. "Increase in Bone Density and Lean Body Mass During Testosterone Administration in Men with Acquired Hypogonadism." *Journal of Clinical Endocrinology and Metabolism* 81(12): 4358–65 (Dec. 1996).

Marin, P., et al. "Assimilation of Triglycerides in Subcutaneous and Intraabdominal Adipose Tissues in Vivo in Men: Effects of Testosterone." *Journal of Clinical Endocrinology and Metabolism* 81(3): 1018–22 (March 1996).

Marin P., B. Oden, and P. Bjorntorp. "Assimilation and Mobilization of Triglycerides in Subcutaneous Abdominal and Femoral Adipose Tissue In Vivo in Men: Effects of Androgens." *Journal of Clinical Endocrinology and Metabolism* 79(5): 1310–06 (Nov. 1994).

Morales, A., et al. "Testosterone Supplementation for Hypogonadal Impotence: Assessment of Biochemical Measures and Therapeutic Outcomes." *Journal of Urology* 157(3): 849–54 (March 1997).

Reid, I. R., et al. "Testosterone Therapy in Glucocorticoid-Treated Men." *Archives of Internal Medicine* 156(11): 1173–77 (June 10, 1996).

Simon, D., et al. "Association Between Plasma Total Testosterone and Cardiovascular Risk Factors in Healthy Adult Men: The Telecom Study." *Journal of Clinical Endocrinology and Metabolism* 82(2): 682–85 (Feb. 1997).

Tibblin, G., et al. "The Pituitary-Gonadal Axis and Health in Elderly Men: A Study of Men Born in 1913." *Diabetes* 45 (11): 1605–09 (Nov. 1996).

Vasquez-Pereyra, F., et al. "Modulation of Short Term and Long Term Memory by Steroid Sexual Hormones." *Life Sciences* 56(14): PL255–PL260 (1995).

Veldhuis, J. D., et al. "Differential Impact of Age, Sex Steroid Hormones, and Obesity on Basal versus Pulsatile Growth Hormone Secretion in Men as Assessed in an Ultrasensitive Chemiluminescence Assay." *Journal of Clinical Endocrinology and Metabolism* 80(11): 3209–22 (Nov. 1995).

Wang, C., et al. "Sublingual Testosterone Replacement Improves Muscle Mass and Strength, Decreases Bone Resorption, and Increases Bone Formation Markers in Hypogonadal Men—A Clinical Research Center Study." *Journal of Clinical Endocrinology and Metabolism* 81(10): 3654–62 (Oct. 1996).

Wang, C., et al. "Testosterone Replacement Therapy Improves Mood in Hypogonadal Men—A Clinical Research Center Study." *Journal of Clinical Endocrinology and Metabolism* 81(10): 3578–83 (Oct. 1996).

Weissberger, A. J., and K. K. Ho. "Activation of the Somatotropic Axis by Testosterone in Adult Males: Evidence for the Role of Aromatization." *Journal of Clinical Endocrinology and Metabolism* 76(6): 1407–12 (June 1993).

Zmunda, J. M., et al. "Testosterone Decreases Lipoprotein (A) in Men." *American Journal of Cardiology* 77(14): 1244–47 (June 1, 1996).

DHEA

Araneo, B., and R. Daynes. "Dehydroepiandosterone Functions as More Than an Antiglucocorticoid in Preserving Immunocompetence After Thermal Injury." *Endocrinology* 136(2): 393–401 (Feb. 1995).

Assan, R., et al. "Dehydroepiandosterone (DHEA) for Diabetic Patients?" *European Journal of Endocrinology* 135: 37–38 (1996).

Barrett-Connor, E., and A. Ferrara. "Dehydroepiandosterone, Dehydroepiandosterone Sulfate, Obesity, Waist-Hip Ratio, and Noninsulin-Dependent Diabetes in Postmenopausal Women: The Rancho Bernardo Study." *Journal of Clinical Endocrinology and Metabolism* 81(1): 59–64 (Jan. 1996).

Baulieu, E. E. "Dehydroepiandrosterone (DHEA): A Fountain of Youth?" *Journal of Clinical Endocrinology and Metabolism* 81(9): 3147–51 (1996).

Beer, N. A., et al. "Dehydroepiandrosterone Reduces Plasma Plasminogen Activator Inhibitor Type 1 and Tissue Plasminogen Activator Antigen in Man." *American Journal of the Medical Sciences* 311(5): 205–10 (May 1996).

Daynes, R., and B. A. Araneo. "The Development of Effective Vaccine Adjuvants Employing Natural Regulators of T-Cell Lymphokine Production In Vivo." *Annals of the New York Academy of Sciences* 730: 144–61 (Aug. 15, 1994).

Eich, D. M., et al. "Inhibition of Accelerated Coronary Atherosclerosis with Dehydroepiandrosterone in the Heterotropic Rabbit Model of Cardiac Transplantation." *Circulation* 87(1): 261–69 (Jan. 1993).

Friess, E., et al. "DHEA Administration Increases Rapid Eye Movement Sleep and EEG Power and Sigma Frequency Range." *American Journal of Physiology* 268: E107–E113 (1995).

Haffner, S. M., and R. A. Valdez. "Endogenous Sex Hormones: Impact on Lipids, Lipoproteins, and Insulin." *American Journal of Medicine* 98(1A): 40S–47S (Jan. 16, 1995).

Herbert, J., et al. "The Age of Dehydroepiandrosterone." *The Lancet* 345: 1193–94 (May 13, 1995).

McLachlan, J. A., C. D. Serkin, and O. Bokouche. "Dehydroepiandrosterone Modulation of Lipopolysaccharide-Stimulated Monocyte Cytotoxity." *Journal of Immunology* 156(1): 328–35 (Jan. 1, 1996).

Morales, A. J., et al. "Effects of Replacement Dose of Dehydroepiandosterone in Men and Women of Advancing Age." *Journal of Clinical Endocrinology and Metabolism* 78: 1360–67 (1994).

Padgett, D. A., and R. M. Loria. "In Vitro Potentiation of Lymphocyte Activation by Dehydroepiandosterone, Androstenediol, and Androstenetriol." *Journal of Immunology* 153(4): 1544–52 (Aug. 15, 1994).

Skolnick, A. A. "Scientific Verdict Still Out on DHEA." *JAMA* 276(17): 1365–67 (Nov. 6, 1996).

Toshiyuki, H., M.D., Ph.D., et al. "Effect of Dehydroepiandosterone Sulfate on Ophthalmic Artery Flow Velocity Wave Forms in Full-Term Pregnant Women." *American Journal of Perinatology* 12(2): 135–37 (March 1995).

Yen, S. S., A. J. Morales, and O. Khorram. "Replacement of DHEA in Aging Men and Women: Potential Remedial Effects." *Annual Report of the N.Y. Academy of Sciences* 774: 128–42 (1995).

PREGNENOLONE

Akwa, Y., and J. Young, et al. "Neurosteroids: Biosynthesis, Metabolism and Function of Pregnenolone and Dehydroepiandosterone in the Brain." *Journal of Steroid Biochemistry* 13(8): 961–63 (1980).

DeWied, D. "Hormone Influences on Motivation, Learning and Memory Processes." *Hospital Practice* 11(1): 123–31 (1976).

———. "Pituitary Adrenal System Hormones and Behavior." *Acta Endocrinologica* 85, Suppl 214: 9–18 (1977).

Flood, J. F., J. E. Morley, and E. Roberts. "Memory-Enhancing Effects in Male Mice of Pregnenolone and Steroids Metabolically Derived from It." *Proceedings of the National Academy of Sciences* 89(5): 1567–71 (1992).

Guth, L., Z. Zhang, and E. Roberts. "Key Role for Pregnenolone in Combination Therapy That Promotes Recovery After Spinal Cord Injury." *Proceedings of the National Academy of Sciences USA* 91(23): 12308–12 (Dec. 6, 1994).

Morfin, R., and G. Courchay. "Pregnenolone and Dehydroepiandosterone as Precursors of Native 7-Hydroxylated Metabolites Which Increase the Immune Response in Mice." *Journal of Steroid Biochemistry and Molecular Biology* 50(1–2): 91–100 (July 1994).

Morfin, R., J. Young, et al. "Neurosteroids: Pregnenolone in Human Sciatic Nerves." *Proceedings of the National Academy of Sciences USA* 9(15): 6790–93 (1992).

Paul, S. M., and R. H. Purdy. "Neuroactive Steroids," *FASEB Journal* 6(6): 2311–22 (1992).

Robel, P., et al. "Biosynthesis and Assay of Neurosteroids in Rats and Mice: Functional Correlates." *Journal of Steroid Biochemistry and Molecular Biology* 53(1–6): 355–60 (June 1995).

Weidenfeld, J., R. A. Siegel, and I. Chowers. "In Vitro Conversion of Pregnenolone to Progesterone by Discrete Brain Areas of the Male Rat." *Journal of Steroid Biochemistry* 13(8): 961–63 (1980).

Wu, F. S., et al. "Pregnenolone Sulfate: A Positive Allosteric Modulator at the N-Methyl-D-Aspartate Receptor." *Molecular Pharmacology* 40(3): 333–36 (1991).

ANDROSTENEDIONE

Mateo, L., et al. "Sex Hormone Status and Bone Mineral Density in Men with Rheumatoid Arthritis." *Journal of Rheumatology* 22(8): 1455–60 (Aug. 1995).

Schweikert, H. U., L. Wolf, and G. Romalo. "Estrogen Formation from Androstenedione in Human Bone." *Clinical Endocrinology* 43(1): 37–42 (July 1995).

CORTISOL

Gotthardt, U., et al. "Cortisol, ACTH, and Cardiovascular Response to a Cognitive Challenge Paradigm in Aging and Depression." *American Journal of Physiology* 268(4 Pt 2): R865–73 (April 1995).

Kern, W., et al. "Changes in Cortisol and Growth Hormone Secretion During Nocturnal Sleep in the Course of Aging." *Journals Gerontology,* Series A, *Biological Sciences and Medical Sciences* 51(1): M3–9 (Jan. 1996).

Lupien, S., et al. "Basal Cortisol Levels and Cognitive Deficits in Human Aging." *Journal of Neuroscience* 14(5 Pt 1): 2893–903 (May 1994).

Nicolson, N., et al. "Salivary Cortisol Levels and Stress Reactivity in Human Aging." *Journals of Gerontology,* Series A, *Biological Sciences and Medical Sciences* 52(2): M68–75 (March 1997).

Stokes, P. E. "The Potential Role of Excessive Cortisol Induced by HPA Hyperfunction in the Pathogenesis of Depression." *European Neuropsychopharmacology* 5, Suppl: 77–82 (1995).

Van Cauter, E., R. Leproult, and D. J. Kupfer. "Effects of Gender and Age on the Levels and Circadian Rhythmicity of Plasma Cortisol." *Journal of Clinical Endocrinology and Metabolism* 81(7): 2468–73 (July 1996).

Wilkinson, C. W., E. R. Peskind, and M. A. Raskind. "Decreased Hypothalamic-Pituitary-Adrenal Axis Sensitivity to Cortisol Feedback Inhibition in Human Aging." *Neuroendocrinology* 65(1): 79–90 (Jan. 1997).

XENOESTROGENS

Colborn, T., F. S. vom Saal, and A. M. Soto. "Developmental Effects of Endocrine-Disrupting Chemicals in Wildlife and Humans." *Environmental Health Perspectives* 101(5): 378–84 (Oct. 1993).

Daston, G. P., et al. "Environmental Estrogens and Reproductive Health: A Discussion of the Human and Environmental Data." *Reproductive Toxicology* 11(4): 465–81 (July 1997).

Sharpe, R. M., et al. "Gestational and Lactational Exposure of Rats to Xenoestrogens Results in Reduced Testicular Size and Sperm Production." *Environmental Health Perspectives* 103(12): 1136–42 (Dec. 1995).

Toppari, J., et al. "Male Reproductive Health and Environmental Xenoestrogens." *Environmental Health Perspectives* 104, Suppl 4: 741–803 (Aug. 1996).

CHAPTER 4:
THE ANTI-AGING HORMONES

GROWTH HORMONE

Angelin, B., and M. Rudling. "Growth Hormone and Hepatic Lipoprotein Metabolism." *Current Opinion in Lipidology* 5(3): 160–65 (June 1994).

Bjorntorp, P. "Endocrine Abnormalities of Obesity." *Metabolism: Clinical and Experimental* 44(9, Suppl 3): 21–23 (Sept. 1995).

Bondy, C. A., et al. "Clinical Uses of Insulin-Like Growth Factor I." *Annals of Internal Medicine* 120(7): 593–601 (April 1, 1994).

Braverman, E. R., et al. *The Healing Nutrients Within.* New Canaan, Conn.: Keats Publishing, 1997.

Bucci, L., Ph.D. "Somatotropin (Growth Hormone) Release by Oral Amino Acids and Peptides in the Long-Lived." *Anti-Aging Medical Therapeutics.* Marina del Rey, Calif.: Health Quest Publications, 1997, pp. 36–49.

Caidahl, K., S. Eden, and B. A. Bengtsson. "Cardiovascular and Renal Effects of Growth Hormone." *Clinical Endocrinology* 40(3): 393–400 (March 1994).

Carey, B., and K. Lee. "The Slumber Solution: Researchers Have Discovered a Surprising Secret to Waking Up Refreshed—And Maybe Even Staying Younger." *Health* 10(4): 70–76 (July–Aug. 1996).

Clark, R. G., et al. "Growth Hormone Secretagogues Stimulate the Hypothalamic-Pituitary-Adrenal Axis and Are Diabetogenic in the Zucker Diabetic Fatty Rat." *Endocrinology* 138(10): 4316–23 (Oct. 1997).

Cranton, E. M., and J. P. Frackelton. "Take Control of Your Aging! How Human Growth Hormone Can Reverse Aging." *Alternative Medicine Digest* (1995).

Cuocolo, A., et al. "Improved Left Ventricular Function After Growth Hormone Replacement in Patients with Hypopituitarism: Assessment with Radionuclide Angiography." *European Journal of Nuclear Medicine* 23(4): 390–94 (April 1996).

Duerr, R. L., et al. "Cardiovascular Effects of Insulin-Like Growth Factor-1 and Growth Hormone in Chronic Left Ventricular Failure in the Rat." *Circulation* 93(12): 2188–96 (June 15, 1996).

Etherton, T. D., et al. "Mechanisms by Which Somatotropin Decreases Adipose Tissue Growth." *American Journal of Clinical Nutrition* 58, Suppl 2: 287S–295S (Aug. 1993).

Froesch, E. R., P. D. Zenobi, and M. Hussain. "Metabolic and Therapeutic Effects of Insulin-Like Growth Factor I." *Hormone Research* 42(1–2): 66–71 (1994).

Gebhart, F. "Antiaging, or Just Raging? Some Doctors Believe That Human Growth Hormone Can Reverse the Aging Process." *Insight on the News* 11(31): 33 (Aug. 14, 1995).

Gelato, M. C. "Aging and Immune Function: A Possible Role for Growth Hormone." *Hormone Research* 45(1–2): 46–49 (1996).

Grunfeld, C., et al. "The Acute Effects of Human Growth Hormone Administration on Thyroid Function in Normal Men." *Journal of Clinical Endocrinology and Metabolism* 67: 1111–14 (1988).

Hertoghe, T. H. "Growth Hormone Therapy in Aging Adults." *Anti-Aging Medical Therapeutics*. Marina del Rey, Calif.: Health Quest Publications, 1997, pp. 10–28.

Holloszy, J. O. "Mortality Rate and Longevity of Food-Restricted Rats: A Reevaluation." *Journal of Applied Physiology* 82(2): 399–403 (Feb. 1997).

Hussain, M. A., et al. "Comparison of the Effects of Growth Hormone and Insulin-Like Growth Factor 1 on Substrate Oxidation and on Insulin Sensitivity in Growth Hormone-Deficient Humans." *Journal of Clinical Investigation* 94(3): 1126–33 (Sept. 1994).

Jamieson, James, and L. E. Dorman, M.D. *Growth Hormone: Reversing Human Aging Naturally—The Methuselah Factor.* East Canaan, Conn.: Safe Goods, 1997.

Jorgensen, J. O. L., et al. "Beneficial Effects of Growth Hormone Therapy in Growth Hormone Deficient Adults." *Lancet* 1: 1221–25 (1989).

Kupfer, S. R., et al. "Enhancement of the Anabolic Effects of Growth Hormone and IGF-1 by Use of Both Agents Simultaneously." *Journal of Clinical Investigation* 91(2): 391–96 (1993).

McGauley, G. A., et al. "Psychological Well-Being Before and After Growth Hormone Treatment in Adults with Growth Hormone Deficiency." *Hormone Research* 33, Suppl 4: 52–54 (1990).

Masoro, E. J. "Possible Mechanisms Underlying the Antiaging Actions of Caloric Restriction." *Toxicology and Pathology* 24(6): 738–41 (Nov.–Dec. 1996).

Mauras, N., S. Q. Doi, and J. R. Shapiro. "Recombinant Insulin-Like Growth Factor I, Recombinant Human Growth Hormone, and Sex Steroids: Effects on Markers of Bone Turnover in Humans." *Journal of Clinical Endocrinology and Metabolism* 81(6): 2222–26 (June 1996).

Meling, T. R., and E. S. Nylen. "Growth Hormone Deficiency in Adults: A Review." *American Journal of the Medical Sciences* 311(4): 153–66 (1996).

Melov, S., et al. "Multi-Organ Characterization of Mitochondrial Genomic Rearrangements in Ad Libitum and Caloric Restricted Mice Show Striking Somatic Mitochondrial DNA Rearrangements with Age." *Nucleic Acids Research* 25(5): 974–82 (March 1, 1997).

Papadakis, M. A., et al. "Growth Hormone Replacement in Healthy Older Men Improves Body Composition but Not Functional Ability." *Annals of Internal Medicine* 124(8): 708–9 (April 15, 1996).

Ross, J., Jr., and M. Hongo. "The Role of Hypertrophy and Growth Factors in Heart Failure." *Journal of Cardiac Failure* 2, Suppl 4: S121–28 (Dec. 1996).

Rosen, T., and B. A. Bengtsson. "Premature Mortality Due to Cardiovascular Disease in Hypopituitarism." *Lancet* 336: 285–88 (1990).

Rudman, D., et al. "Effects of Human Growth Hormone in Men over 60 Years Old." *The New England Journal of Medicine* 323: 1–6 (July 5, 1990).

Sahelian, R., "Natural Growth Hormone Releasers." *Let's Live:* 68–72 (June 1997).

Schteingart, D. E., "Suppression of Cortisol Secretion by Human Growth Hormone." *Journal of Clinical Endocrinology and Metabolism* 50: 721–25 (1980).

Schwartz, R. S. "Trophic Factor Supplementation: Effect on the Age-Associated Changes in Body Composition." *Journals of Gerontology,* Series A, *Biological Sciences & Medical Sciences* 50: 151–56 (Nov. 1995).

Shalet, S. M. "Growth Hormone Deficiency and Replacement in Adults: Useful in Those With Reduced Quality of Life or Bone Mineral Density." *British Medical Journal* 313(7053): 314 (Aug. 10, 1996).

Terry, L. C., and E. Chein. "Growth Hormone Therapy in 202 Aging Adults." Unpublished study.

Veldhuis, J. D., et al. "Differential Impact of Age, Sex Steroid Hormones, and Obesity on Basal versus Pulsatile Growth Hormone Secretion in Men as Assessed in an Ultrasensitive Chemiluminescence Assay." *Journal of Clinical Endocrinology and Metabolism* 80(11): 3209–22 (Nov. 1995).

Veldhuis, J. D., et al. "Dual Effects in Pulsatile Growth Hormone Secretion and Clearance Subserve the Hyposomatotropism of Obesity in Men." *Journal of Clinical Endocrinology and Metabolism* 72: 51–59 (1991).

Vermeulen, A., J. M. Kaufman, and V. A. Giagulli. "Influence of Some Biological Indexes on Sex Hormone-Binding Globulin and Androgen Levels in Aging or Obese Males." *Journal of Clinical Endocrinology and Metabolism* 1821–26 (May 1996).

Weindruch, R. "The Retardation of Aging by Caloric Restriction: Studies in Rodents and Primates." *Toxicology and Pathology* 24(6): 742–45 (Nov.–Dec. 1996).

Weltman, A., et al. "Endurance Training Amplifies the Pulsatile Release of Growth Hormone: Effects of Training Intensity." *Journal of Applied Physiology* 72(6): 2188–96 (1992).

Weltman, A., et al. "Exercise Training Decreases the Growth Hormone (GH) Response to Acute Constant-Load Exercise." *Medicine & Science in Sports & Exercise* 29(5): 669–76 (May 1997).

Wit, J. M., et al. "Immunological Findings in Growth Hormone-Treated Patients." *Hormone Research* 39(3–4): 107–10 (1993).

Xu, X., and W. E. Sonntag. "Moderate Caloric Restriction Prevents the Age-Related Decline in Growth Hormone Receptor Signal Transduction." *The Journals of Gerontology* 51(2): B167–68 (1996).

Yamada, M., et al. "The Indirect Participation of Growth Hormone in the Thymocyte Proliferation System." *Cellular & Molecular Biology* 40(2): 111–21 (March 1994).

Yanick, Paul Jr., Ph.D., and Vincent C. Giampapa, M.D. *Quantum Longevity.* San Diego, Calif.: ProMotion Publishing, 1997.

INSULIN

Atkins, R. C., M.D. *Dr. Atkins' New Diet Revolution.* New York: M. Evans and Company, 1992.

Despres, J. P., et al. "Regional Distribution of Body Fat, Plasma Lipoproteins, and Cardiovascular Disease." *Arteriosclerosis* 10: 497–511 (July–Aug. 1990).

"Entering a High-Protein Twilight Zone." *Tufts University Diet and Nutrition Letter* 14(3): 4–6 (May 1996).

Golay, A., et al. "Weight-Loss with Low or High Carbohydrate Diet?" *International Journal of Obesity and Related Metabolic Disorders* 20(12): 1067–72 (Dec. 1996).

Gould, K. L., et al. "Changes in Myocardial Perfusion Abnormalities by Positron Emission Tomography After Long-Term, Intense Risk Factor Modification." *JAMA* 274(11): 894–901 (Sept. 20, 1995).

Jacobs, R. "New Diet, Same Old Snake Oil," *Vegetarian Times* 235: 22 (March 1997).

Kaplan, N. M. "The Deadly Quartet: Upper-Body Obesity, Glucose Intolerance, Hypertriglyceridemia, and Hypertension." *Archives of Internal Medicine* 149: 1514–20 (July 1989).

Marston, W. "The New Diet Food: High-Protein Diets Really Do Make You Lose Fat; That's Where the Problems Start." *Health* 10(5): 98–102 (Sept. 1996).

McCord, H. "Meat, Milk, and Bones." *Prevention* 49(9): 51 (Sept. 1997).

Norris, E. "High-Protein Diets: Where's the Beef?" *Harvard Health Letter* 22(3): 1–3 (Jan. 1997).

Ornish, D. M., et al. "Can Lifestyle Changes Reverse Atherosclerosis?" *Lancet* 336: 129–33 (1990).

Reaven, G. M. "Role of Insulin Resistance in Human Disease." *Diabetes* 37: 1595–1607 (1988).

Plotnick, G. D., M. C. Corretti, and R. A. Vogel. "Effect of Antioxidant Vitamins on the Transient Impairment of Endothelium-Dependent Brachial Artery Vasoactivity Following a Single High-Fat Meal." *JAMA* 278(20): 1682–86 (Nov. 26, 1997).

Thomas, D. "Dangerous Dieting: Weight-Loss Fads Can Be Hazardous to the Health." *Maclean's* 110(6): 54 (Feb. 10, 1997).

MELATONIN

Anisimov, V. N., I. G. Popovich, and M. A. Zabezhinski. "Melatonin and Colon Carcinogenesis: I. Inhibitory Effect of Melatonin on Development of Intestinal Tumors Induced by 1,2-Dimethylhydrazine in Rats." *Carcinogenesis* 18(8): 1549–53 (Aug. 1997).

Brugger, P. "Impaired Nocturnal Secretion of Melatonin in Coronary Heart Disease." *The Lancet* 345: 1408 (June 3, 1995).

Elam, R. P. "Effects of Arginine and Ornithine on Strength, Lean Body Mass, and Urinary Hydroxyproline in Adult Males." *Journal of Sports Medicine* 29: 52–56 (1989).

Escames, G., et al. "Melatonin and Vitamin E Limit Nitric Oxide-Induced Lipid Peroxidation in Rat Brain Homogenates." *Neuroscience Letters* 230(3): 147–50 (July 25, 1997).

Gilad, E. "Melatonin Is a Scavenger of Peroxynitrite." *Life Sciences* 60(10): 169–74 (1997).

Hara, M., et al. "Administration of Melatonin and Related Indoles Prevents Exercise-Induced Cellular Oxidative Changes in Rats." *Biological Signals* 6(2): 90–100 (March–April 1997).

Kelly, M. R., and G. Loo. "Melatonin Inhibits Oxidative Modification of Human Low-Density Lipoprotein." *Journal of Pineal Research* 22(4): 203–9 (May 1997).

Lemus, W. A., et al. "Melatonin Blocks the Stimulatory Effect of Prolactin on Human Breast Cancer Cell Growth in Culture." *British Journal of Cancer* 72: 1435–40 (1995).

Maestroni, G. J., and A. Conti. "Melatonin and the Immune-Hematopoetic System: Therapeutic and Adverse Pharmacological Correlates." *Neuroimmunomodulation* 3(6): 325–32 (Nov.–Dec. 1996).

Magri, F., et al. "Changes in Endocrine Circadian Rhythms as Markers of Physiological and Pathological Brain Aging." *Chronobiology International* 14(4): 385–96 (July 1997).

Monteleone, P., et al. "Physical Exercise at Night Blunts the Nocturnal Increase of Plasma Melatonin Levels in Healthy Humans." *Life Sciences* 47(22): 1989–95 (1990).

Montilla, P., et al. "Hyperlipidemic Nephropathy Induced by Adriamycin: Effect of Melatonin Administration." *Nephron* 76: 345–50 (1997).

Okatani, Y., et al. "Melatonin Inhibits Vasospastic Action of Hydrogen Peroxide in Human Umbilical Artery." *Journal of Pineal Research* 22(3): 163–68 (April 1997).

Palm, L., et al. "Long-Term Melatonin Treatment in Blind Children and Young Adults with Circadian Sleep-Wake Disturbances." *Developmental Medicine and Child Neurology* 39: 319–25 (1997).

Panzer, A., and M. Viljoen. "The Validity of Melatonin as an Oncostatic Agent." *Journal of Pineal Research* 22(4): 184–202 (May 1997).

Pierpaoli, W., W. Regelson, and C. Colman. *The Melatonin Miracle: Nature's Age-Reversing, Disease-Fighting, Sex-Enhancing Hormone.* New York: Simon & Schuster, 1995.

Sahelian, R., M.D. *Melatonin: Nature's Sleeping Pill.* Marina Del Rey, Calif.: Be Happier Press, 1995, p. 5.

Skwarlo-Sonta, K. "Functional Connections Between the Pineal Gland and Immune System." *Acta Neurobiologiae Experimentalis* 56(1): 341–57 (1996).

Wurtman, R. J., and I. Zhdanova. "Improvement of Sleep Quality by Melatonin." *The Lancet* 346: 1491 (Dec. 2, 1995).

CHAPTER 5:
KEEPING CELLS YOUNG BY SQUELCHING OXIDATION

Aomine, M., and M. Arita. "Pretreatment with Coenzyme Q10 Protects Guinea Pig Ventricular Muscle from Hypoxia-Induced Deterioration of Action Potentials and Contraction." *General Pharmacology* 15(2): 91–96 (1985).

Beyer, R. E. "An Analysis of the Role of Coenzyme Q in Free Radical Generation and As an Antioxidant." *Biochemistry and Cell Biology* 70(6): 390–403 (June 1992).

Bliznakov, E. G., and G. L. Hunt. *The Miracle Nutrient: Coenzyme Q10.* New York: Bantam Books, 1989.

Cameron, Ewan, and Linus Pauling. *Cancer and Vitamin C.* Menlo Park, Calif.: The Linus Pauling Institute of Science and Medicine, 1979.

Conner, E. M., and M. B. Grisham. "Inflammation, Free Radicals, and Antioxidants." *Nutrition* 12: 274–77 (1996).

Constantinescu, A., et al. "Alpha-Lipoic Acid Protects Against Hemolysis of Human Erythrocytes Induced by Peroxyl Radicals." *Biochemistry and Molecular Biology International* 33(4): 669–79 (July 1994).

Davies, K. J. "Oxidative Stress: The Paradox of Aerobic Life." *Biochemical Society Symposia* 61: 1–31 (1995).

Dubois-Rende, J. L., et al. "Oxidative Stress in Patients with Unstable Angina." *European Heart Journal* 15: 179–83 (1994).

Florence, T. M. "The Role of Free Radicals in Disease." *Australian and New Zealand Journal of Ophthalmology* 23(1): 3–7 (Feb. 1995).

Gomez-Diaz, C., et al. "Antioxidant Ascorbate is Stabilized by NADH-Coenzyme Q10 Reductase in the Plasma Membrane." *Journal of Bioenergetics and Biomembranes* 29(3): 251–57 (June 1997).

Gorog, P. "Neutrophil-Oxidized Low Density Lipoprotein: Generation in and Clearance from the Plasma." *International Journal of Experimental Pathology* 73(4): 485–90 (Aug. 1992).

Halliwell, B. "Free Radicals, Antioxidants, and Human Disease: Curiosity, Cause, or Consequence?" *The Lancet* 344: 721–24 (Sept. 10, 1994).

———. "Free Radicals and Antioxidants: A Personal View." *Nutrition Reviews* 52(8): 253–65 (Aug. 1994).

Jacob, R. A., and B. J. Burri. "Oxidative Damage and Defense." *American Journal of Clinical Nutrition* 63(6): 985S–990S (June 1996).

Kanter, M. "Free Radicals, Exercise, and Antioxidant Supplementation." *International Journal of Sports Nutrition* 4: 205–20 (1994).

Kontoghiorghes, G. J., and E. D. Weinberg. "Iron: Mammalian Defense Systems, Mechanisms of Disease, and Chelation Therapy Approaches." *Blood Reviews* 9(1): 33–45 (March 1995).

Kubow, S. "Routes of Formation and Toxic Consequences of Lipid Oxidation Products in Foods." *Free Radical Biology and Medicine* 12(1): 63–81 (1992).

Littarru, G. P., et al. "Metabolic Implications of Coenzyme Q10 in Red Blood Cells and Plasma Lipoproteins." *Molecular Aspects of Medicine* 15, Suppl: s67–72 (1994).

McCord, J. M. "Effects of Positive Iron Status at a Cellular Level." *Nutrition Reviews* 54(3): 85–88 (March 1996).

Nappi, A. J., and E. Vass. "Comparative Studies of Enhanced Iron-Mediated Production of Hydroxyl Radical by Glutathione, Cysteine, Ascorbic Acid, and Selected Catechols." *Biochimica Biophysica Acta* 1336(2): 295–302 (Aug. 29, 1997).

O'Keefe, J. H., Jr., C. J. Lavie, Jr., and B. D. McCallister. "Insights into the Pathogenesis and Prevention of Coronary Artery Disease." *Mayo Clinic Proceedings* 70(1): 69–79 (Jan. 1995).

Reiter, R. J. "Oxygen Radical Detoxification Processes During Aging: The Functional Importance of Melatonin." *Aging* 7(5): 340–51 (Oct. 1995).

Reiter, R. J. "The Pineal Gland and Melatonin in Relation to Aging: A Summary of the Theories and of the Data." *Experimental Gerontology* 30(3–4): 199–212 (May–Aug. 1995).

Rojas, C., et al. "Effect of Vitamin C on Antioxidants, Lipid Peroxidation, and GSH System in the Normal Guinea Pig Heart." *Journal of Nutritional Science and Vitaminology* 40: 411–20 (1994).

Sies, H., and W. Stahl. "Vitamins E, C, Beta-Carotene, and Other Carotenoids as Antioxidants." *American Journal of Clinical Nutrition* 62, Suppl 6: 1315S–1321S (Dec. 1995).

Sinatra, S. T., and J. DeMarco. "Free Radicals, Oxidative Stress, Oxidized Low Density Lipoprotein, and the Heart: Antioxidants and Other Strategies to Limit Cardiovascular Damage." *Connecticut Medicine* 59(10): 579–88 (Oct. 1995).

Sullivan, J. L., "Iron versus Cholesterol—Perspectives on the Iron and Heart Disease Debate." *Journal of Clinical Epidemiology* 49(12): 1345–52 (Dec. 1996).

Thomas, S. R., et al. "Coantioxidants Make Alpha-Tocopherol an Efficient Antioxidant for Low-Density Lipoprotein." *American Journal of Clinical Nutrition* 62, Suppl 6: 1357S–1364S (Dec. 1995).

Wurzelmann, J. I., et al. "Iron Intake and the Risk of Colorectal Cancer." *Cancer Epidemiology and Biomarkers* 5(7): 503–7 (July 1996).

CHAPTER 6:
MAINTAINING MUSCLE FOR LIFE

Armsey, T. J., Jr., and G. A. Green. "Nutritional Supplements: Science vs. Hype." *The Physician and Sportsmedicine* 25(6): 77–92, 116 (June 1997).

Balsom, P. D., K. Soderlund, and B. Ekblom. "Creatine in Humans with Special Reference to Creatine Supplementation." *Sports Medicine* 18(4): 268–80 (Oct. 1994).

Bhasin, S., et al. "The Effects of Supraphysiologic Doses of Testosterone on Muscle Size and Strength in Normal Men." *New England Journal of Medicine* 335(1): 1–7 (July 4, 1996).

Black, V. H. "Intraadrenal Steroid Metabolism in the Guinea Pig." *Endocrine Research* 21: 28–35 (Feb.–May 1995).

Bliznakov, Emil G., and Gerald L. Hunt. *The Miracle Nutrient: Coenzyme Q10.* New York: Bantam Books, 1989.

Brodsky, I. G., P. Balagopal, and K. S. Nair. "Effects of Testosterone Replacement on Muscle Mass and Muscle Protein Synthesis in Hypogonadal Men—A Clinical Research Study." *Journal of Clinical Endocrinology and Metabolism* 81(10): 3469–75 (Oct. 1996).

Campbell, W. W., et al. "Increased Energy Requirements and Changes in Body Composition with Resistance Training in Older Adults." *American Journal of Clinical Nutrition* 60(2): 167–75 (Aug. 1994).

Castaneda, C., et al. "Protein Turnover and Energy Metabolism of Elderly Women Fed a Low-Protein Diet." *American Journal of Clinical Nutrition* 62(1): 40–48 (July 1995).

Clarkson, P. M. "Nutrition for Improved Sports Performance: Current Issues on Ergogenic Aids." *Sports Medicine* 21(6): 393–401 (June 1996).

Eakman, G. D., et al. "The Effects of Testosterone and Dihydrotestosterone on Hypothalamic Regulation of Growth Hormone Secretion." *Journal of Clinical Endocrinology and Metabolism* 81(3): 1217–23 (March 1996).

Evans, W. J. "Exercise, Nutrition, and Aging." *Clinics in Geriatric Medicine* 11(4): 725–34 (Nov. 1995).

Fielding, R. A. "Effects of Exercise in the Elderly: Impact of Progressive-Resistance Training on Skeletal Muscle and Whole-Body Protein Metabolism." *Proceedings of the Nutrition Society* 54(3): 665–75 (Nov. 1996).

Foster, Stephen. "Ginseng Gets to the Root of Health." *Better Nutrition for Today's Living* 66–69 (March 1995).

Giustina, A., et al. "Maturation of the Regulation of Growth Hormone Secretion in Young Males with Hypogonadotropic Hypogonadism Pharmacologically Exposed to Progressive Increments in Serum Testosterone." *Journal of Clinical Endocrinology and Metabolism* 82(4): 1210–19 (April 1997).

Green, James. *The Male Herbal: Health Care for Men and Boys.* Freedom, Calif.: The Crossing Press, 1991.

Kido, Y., et al. "Japanese Dietary Protein Allowance Is Sufficient for Moderate Physical Exercise in Young Men." *Journal of Nutritional Science & Vitaminology* 43(1): 59–71 (Feb. 1997).

Klatz, Ronald, and Carol Kahn. *Grow Young with HGH.* New York: HarperCollins Publishers, 1997.

Kraemer, W. J., et al. "Endogenous Anabolic Hormonal and Growth Factor Responses to Heavy Resistance Exercise in Males and Females." *International Journal of Sports Medicine* 12: 228–35 (1991).

Kreider, R. B., V. Miriel, and E. Bertun. "Amino Acid Supplementation and Exercise Performance. Analysis of the Proposed Ergogenic Value." *Sports Medicine* 16(3): 190–209 (Sept. 1993).

Lampman, R. M. "Exercise Prescription for Chronically Ill Patients." *American Family Physician* 55(6): 2185–92 (May 1, 1997).

MacLean, D. A., T. E. Graham, and B. Saltin. "Stimulation of Muscle Ammonia Production During Exercise Following Branched-Chain Amino Acid Supplementation in Humans." *Journal of Physiology* 493(Pt 3): 909–22 (June 15, 1996).

Maughan, R. J., et al. "Diet Composition and the Performance of High-Intensity Exercise." *Journal of Sports Sciences* 15(3): 265–75 (June 1997).

Morales, A. J., et al. "Effects of Replacement Dose of Dehydroepiandosterone in Men and Women of Advancing Age." *Journal of Clinical Endocrinology and Metabolism* 78: 1360–67 (1994).

Physical Activity and Health: A Report of the Surgeon General. Centers for Disease Control, July 11, 1996.

Rimar, S., et al. "Pulmonary Protective and Vasodilator Effects of a Standardized Panax Ginseng Preparation Following Artificial Gastric Digestion." *Pulmonary Pharmacology* 9: 205–9 (1996).

Sahelian, Ray, M.D. "Creatine: Nature's Muscle Builder." *Let's Live:* 104 (March 1997).

Suminski, R. R., et al. "Acute Effect of Amino Acid Ingestion and Resistance Exercise on Plasma Growth Hormone Concentration in Young Men." *International Journal of Sport Nutrition* 7: 48–60 (1997).

Turner, Lisa. "Ginseng's Benefits Are Well Rooted." *Vitamin Retailer:* 46–52 (March 1996).

Veldhuis, J. D., et al. "Differential Impact of Age, Sex Steroid Hormones, and Obesity on Basal versus Pulsatile Growth Hormone Secretion in Men As Assessed in an Ultrasensitive Chemiluminescence Assay." *Journal of Clinical Endocrinology and Metabolism* 80(11): 3209–22 (Nov. 1995).

Volek, J. S. "Testosterone and Cortisol in Relationship to Dietary Nutrients and Resistance Exercise." *Journal of Applied Physiology* 82(1): 49–54 (Jan. 1997).

Volek, J. S., et al. "Creatine Supplementation Enhances Muscular Performance During High-Intensity Resistance Exercise." *Journal of the American Dietetic Association* 97: 765–70 (1997).

Wang, C., et al. "Sublingual Testosterone Replacement Improves Muscle Mass and Strength, Decreases Bone Resorption, and Increases Bone Formation Markers in Hypogonadal Men—A Clinical Research Center Study." *Journal of Clinical Endocrinology and Metabolism* 81(10): 3654–62 (Oct. 1996).

Weltman, A., et al. "Endurance Training Amplifies the Pulsatile Release of Growth Hormone: Effects of Training Intensity." *Journal of Applied Physiology* 72(6): 2188–96 (1992).

Yen, S. S., A. J. Morales, and O. Khorram. "Replacement of DHEA in Aging Men and Women: Potential Remedial Effects." *Annals of the New York Academy of Sciences* 774: 128–42 (1995).

CHAPTER 7:
KEEPING UP IN THE BEDROOM

Andersson, S. O., et al. "Body Size and Prostate Cancer: A 20-Year Follow-Up Study Among 135,006 Swedish Construction Workers." *Journal of the National Cancer Institute* 89(5): 385–89 (March 5, 1997).

Arver, S., et al. "Improvement of Sexual Function in Testosterone Deficient Men Treated for One Year with a Permeation Enhanced Testosterone Transdermal System." *Journal of Urology* 155(5): 1604–8 (May 1996).

Azadzoi, K. M., and I. Saenz de Tejada. "Hypercholesterolemia Impairs Endothelium-Dependent Relaxation of Rabbit Corpus Cavernosum Smooth Muscle." *Journal of Urology* 146(1): 238–40 (July 1991).

Bush, P. A., et al. "Nitric Oxide Is a Potent Relaxant of Human and Rabbit Corpus Cavernosum." *Journal of Urology* 147(6): 1650–55 (June 1992).

Choi, H. K., D. H. Seong, and K. H. Rha. "Clinical Efficacy of Korean Red Ginseng for Erectile Dysfunction." *International Journal of Impotence Research* 7(3): 181–86 (Sept. 1995).

DePalma, R. G. "New Developments in Diagnosis and Treatment of Impotence." *Western Journal of Medicine* 164(1): 54–61 (Jan. 1996).

Dunsmuir, W. D., and S. A. Holmes. "The Aetiology and Management of Erectile, Ejaculatory, and Fertility Problems in Men with Diabetes Mellitus." *Diabetes Medicine* 13(8): 700–708 (Aug. 1996).

Green, J. *The Male Herbal.* Freedom, Calif.: The Crossing Press, 1991.

Harrison, P. T., P. Holmes, and C. D. Humfrey. "Reproductive Health in Humans and Wildlife: Are Adverse Trends Associated with Environmental Chemical Exposure?" *Sci. Total Environ.* 205(2–3): 97–106 (Oct. 20, 1997).

Heller, J. E., and P. Gleich. "Erectile Impotence: Evaluation and Management." *Journal of Family Practice* 26(3): 321–24 (March 1988).

Jensen, T. K., et al. "Do Environmental Estrogens Contribute to the Decline in Male Reproductive Health?" *Clinical Chemistry* 41(12 Pt 2): 1896–901 (Dec. 1995).

Leland, J. "A Pill for Impotence?" *Newsweek:* 62–68 (Nov. 17, 1997).

Maatman, T. J., D. K. Montague, and L. M. Martin. "Erectile Dysfunction in Men with Diabetes Mellitus." *Urology:* 589–92 (June 1987).

Michal, V. "Arterial Disease As a Cause of Impotence." *Clinical Endocrinology and Metabolism* 11(3): 725–48 (Nov. 1982).

Montague, D. K., et al. "Clinical Guidelines Panel on Erectile Dysfunction: Summary Report on the Treatment of Organic Erectile Dysfunction." *Journal of Urology* 156(6): 2007–11 (Dec. 1996).

Morales, A., et al. "Testosterone Supplementation for Hypogonadal Impotence: Assessment of Biochemical Measures and Therapeutic Outcomes." *Journal of Urology* 157(3): 849–54 (March 1997).

O'Keefe, M., and D. K. Hunt. "Assessment and Treatment of Impotence." *Medical Clinics of North America* 79(2): 415–34 (March 1995).

Paick, J. S., and J. H. Lee. "An Experimental Study of the Effect of Ginkgo Biloba Extract on the Human and Rabbit Corpus Cavernosum Tissue." *Journal of Urology* 156(5): 1876–80 (Nov. 1996).

Pasquali, R., et al. "Weight Loss and Sex Steroid Metabolism in Massively Obese Man." *Journal of Endocrinology Investigation* 11(3): 205–10 (March 1988).

Schiavi, R. C., et al. "Effect of Testosterone Administration on Sexual Behavior and Mood in Men with Erectile Dysfunction." *Archives of Sexual Behavior* 26(3): 231–41 (June 1997).

Sharpe, R. M., et al. "Gestational and Lactational Exposure of Rats to Xenoestrogens Results in Reduced Testicular Size and Sperm Production." *Environmental Health Perspectives* 103: 1136–43 (1995).

Tanagho, E. A., and J. W. McAninch, eds. *Smith's General Urology.* Norwalk, Conn.: Appleton and Lange, 1992.

Toppari, J., et al. "Male Reproductive Health and Environmental Xenoestrogens." *Environmental Health Perspectives* 104, Suppl 4: 741–803 (Aug. 1996).

Vogt, H. J., et al. "Double-Blind, Placebo-Controlled Safety and Efficacy Trial with Yohimbine Hydrochloride in the Treatment of Nonorganic Erectile Dysfunction." *International Journal of Impotence Research* 9(3): 155–61 (Sept. 1997).

Wabrek, A. J. "Sexual Dysfunction Associated with Diabetes Mellitus." *Journal of Family Practice* 8(4): 735–40 (April 1979).

CHAPTER 8:
PROTECTING YOUR PROSTATE

Adolfsson, J., G. Steineck, and P. O. Hedlund. "Deferred Treatment of Clinically Localized Low-Grade Prostate Cancer: Actual 10-Year and Projected 15-Year Follow-Up of the Karolinska Series." *Urology* 50(5): 722–26 (Nov. 1997).

Albertsen, P. C. "Screening for Prostate Cancer is Neither Appropriate nor Cost-Effective." *Urology Clinics of North America* 23(4): 521–30 (Nov. 1996).

Barasch, M. I. "The Amazing Power of Visualization." *Natural Health* 64 (July–Aug. 1994).

Berges, R. R., et al. "Randomised, Placebo-Controlled, Double-Blind Critical Trial of Beta-Sitosterol in Patients with Benign Prostatic Hyperplasia." *Lancet* 345(8964): 1529–32 (June 17, 1995).

Brawley, O. W. "Prostate Carcinoma Incidence and Patient Mortality: The Effects of Screening and Early Detection." *Cancer* 80(9): 1857–63 (Nov. 1, 1997).

Brown, D. "European Phytomedicines: Research Updates on Chemistry, Pharmacology, and Clinical Applications." *Quarterly Review of Natural Medicine:* 23–29 (Spring 1997).

Chodak, G. W., and H. W. Schoenberg. "Progress and Problems in Screening for Carcinoma of the Prostate." *World Journal of Surgery* 13: 60 (1989).

Clinton, S. K., et al. "Dietary Fat and Protein Intake Differ in Modulation of Prostate Tumor Growth, Prolactin Secretion and Metabolism, and Prostate Gland Prolactin Binding Capacity in Rats." *Journal of Nutrition* 127(2): 225–37 (Feb. 1997).

Daviglus, M. L., et al. "Dietary Beta-Carotene, Vitamin C, and Risk of Prostate Cancer: Results from the Western Electric Study." *Epidemiology* 7(5): 472–77 (Sept. 1996).

de Lignieres, B. "Transdermal Dihydrotestosterone Treatment of 'Andropause'." *Annals of Medicine* 25(3): 235–41 (June, 1993).

Ding, V. D., et al. "Sex Hormone-Binding Globulin Mediates Prostate Androgen Receptor Action via a Novel Signaling Pathway." *Endocrinology* 139(1): 213–18 (Jan. 1998).

Dolby, V. "Scientific Review: Nutritional Supplements and Remedies for Men." *Vitamin Retailer:* 39–42 (Jan. 1998).

Ekman, P. "Endocrine Therapy for Benign Prostatic Hypertrophy in the '90s." *Journal d'Urologie* 101(1): 22–25 (1995).

Farnsworth, W. E. "Role of Estrogen and SHBG in Prostate Physiology." *Prostate* 28(1): 17–23 (Jan. 1996).

Geller, J., et al. "Therapeutic Controversies: Clinical Treatment of Benign Prostatic Hyperplasia." *Journal of Clinical Endocrinology and Metabolism* 80(3): 745–47 (March 1995).

Giovannucci, E., et al. "Intake of Carotenoids and Retinol in Relation to Risk of Prostate Cancer." *Journal of the National Cancer Institute* 687(23): 1767–76 (Dec. 1995).

Golan, R. *Optimal Wellness.* New York: Ballantine Books, 1995.

Habenicht, U. F., et al. "Management of Benign Prostatic Hyperplasia with Particular Emphasis on Aromatase Inhibitors." *Journal of Steroid Biochemistry and Molecular Biology* 44(4–6): 557–63 (March 1993).

Hall, A. K. "Liarozole Amplifies Retinoid-Induced Apoptosis in Human Prostate Cancer Cells." *Anti-Cancer Drugs* 7(3): 312–20 (May 1996).

Hartman, R. W., M. Mark, and F. Soldati. "Inhibition of 5-Alpha-Reductase and Aromatase by PHL-00801 (Prostatonin), a Combination of PY 102 *(Pygeum africanum)* and UR 102 *(Urtica dioica)* Extracts." *Phytomedicine* 3(2): 121–28 (1996).

Klippel, K. P., D. M. Hiltl, and B. Schipp. "A Multicentric, Placebo-Controlled, Double-Blind Clinical Trial of Beta-Sitosterol (Phytosterol) for the Treatment of Benign Prostatic Hyperplasia." *British Journal of Urology* 80: 427–32 (1997).

Kolonel, L. N. "Nutrition and Prostate Cancer." *Cancer Causes and Control* 7(1): 83–144 (Jan. 1996).

Lissoni, P., M. Cazzaniga, G. Tancini, et al. "Reversal of Clinical Resistance to LHRH Analogue in Metastatic Prostate Cancer by the Pineal Hormone Melatonin: Efficacy of LHRH Analogue plus Melatonin in Patients Progressing on LHRH Analogue Alone." *European Urology* 31: 178–81 (1997).

Littrup, P. J. "Future Benefits and Cost-Effectiveness of Prostate Carcinoma Screening." *Cancer* 80(9): 1864–70 (Nov. 1, 1997).

Lowe, F. C., and J. C. Ku. "Phytotherapy in Treatment of Benign Prostatic Hyperplasia: A Critical Review." *Urology* 48(1): 12–20 (July 1996).

Magoha, G. A. "Medical Management of Benign Prostatic Hyperplasia: A Review." *East African Medical Journal* 73(7): 453–56 (July 1996).

Makela, S. I., et al. "Dietary Soybean May Be Antiestrogenic in Male Mice." *Journal of Nutrition* 125(3): 437–45 (March 1995).

McConnell, J. D. "Benign Prostatic Hyperplasia. Hormonal Treatment." *Urologic Clinics of North America* 22(2): 387–400 (May 1995).

Mettlin, C. J., et al. "Results of Hospital Cancer Registry Surveys by the American College of Surgeons: Outcome of Prostate Cancer Treatment by Radical Prostatectomy." *Cancer* 80(9): 1875–81 (Nov. 1, 1997).

Metzker, H., M. Kieser, and U. Holscher. "Efficacy of a Combined *Sabal-Urtica* Preparation in the Treatment of Benign Prostatic Hyperplasia." *Urologe* [B] 36: 292–300 (1996).

Murray, M., and J. Pizzorno. *Encyclopedia of Natural Medicine.* Rocklin, Calif.: Prima Publishing, 1991.

Nag, S., et al. "Transperineal Palladium 103 Prostate Brachytherapy: Analysis of Morbidity and Seed Migration." *Urology* 45(1): 87–92 (Jan. 1995).

Nakhla, A. M., N. A. Romas, and W. Rosner. "Estradiol Activates the Prostate Androgen Receptor and Prostate-Specific Antigen Secretion Through the Intermediacy of Sex Hormone-Binding Globulin." *Journal of Biological Chemistry* 272(11): 6838–41 (March 14, 1997).

Nakhla, A. M., et al. "Estradiol Causes the Rapid Accumulation of cAMP in Human Prostate." *Proceedings of the National Academy of Sciences of the United States of America* 91(12): 5402–5 (June 7, 1994).

Newcomer, L. M., et al. "Temporal Trends in Rates of Prostate Cancer: Declining Incidence of Advanced Stage Disease, 1974 to 1994." *Journal of Urology* 158(4): 1427–30 (Oct. 1997).

Pollard, M., and P. H. Luckert. "Influence of Isoflavones in Soy Protein Isolates on Development of Induced Prostate-Related Cancers in L-W Rats." *Nutrition and Cancer* 28(1): 41–45 (1997).

Randall, V. A. "Role of 5-Alpha-Reductase in Health and Disease." *Baillieres Clinical Endocrinology & Metabolism* 8(2): 405–31 (April 1994).

Rittmaster, R. S. "Finasteride." *New England Journal of Medicine* 330(2): 120–25 (Jan. 13, 1994).

Rose, D. P. "Effects of Dietary Fatty Acids on Breast and Prostate Cancers: Evidence from In Vitro Experiments and Animal Studies." *American Journal of Clinical Nutrition* 66, Suppl 6: 1513S–1522S (Dec. 1997).

Santti, R., et al. "Developmental Estrogenization and Prostatic Neoplasia." *Prostate* 24(2): 67–78 (1994).

Sigounas, G., A. Anagnostou, and M. Steiner. "dl-Alpha-Tocopherol Induces Apoptosis in Erythroleukemia, Prostate, and Breast Cancer Cells." *Nutrition and Cancer* 28(1): 30–35 (1997).

Siiteri, P. K., J. D. Wilson, and J. A. Mayfield. "The Formation and Content of Dihydrotestosterone in the Hypertrophic Prostate of Man." *The Journal of Clinical Investigation* 49: 1737–45 (1970).

Smart, C. R. "The Results of Prostate Carcinoma Screening in the U.S. As Reflected by the Surveillance, Epidemiology, and End Results Program." *Cancer* 80(9): 1835–44, (Nov. 1, 1997).

Steers, W. D., and B. Zorn. "Benign Prostatic Hyperplasia." *Disease-A-Month* 41(7): 437–97 (July 1995).

Walsh, Patrick, M.D., and Janet Farrar Worthington. *The Prostate: A Guide for Men and the Women Who Love Them.* Baltimore: The Johns Hopkins University Press, 1995.

Wennbo, H., et al. "Transgenic Mice Overexpressing the Prolactin Gene Develop Dramatic Enlargement of the Prostate Gland." *Endocrinology* 138(10): 4410–15 (Oct. 1997).

Whittemore, A. S., et al. "Prostate Cancer in Relation to Diet, Physical Activity, and Body Size in Blacks, Whites, and Asians in the United States and Canada." *Journal of the National Cancer Institute* 87(9): 652–61 (May 3, 1995).

Willett, W. C. "Specific Fatty Acids and Risks of Breast and Prostate Cancer: Dietary Intake." *American Journal of Clinical Nutrition* 66, Suppl 6: 1557S–1563S (Dec. 1997).

Woolf, S. H. "Screening for Prostate Cancer with Prostate-Specific Antigen. An Examination of the Evidence." *New England Journal of Medicine* 333(21): 1401–5 (Nov. 23, 1995).

Yip, I., W. Aronson, and D. Heber. "Nutritional Approaches to the Prevention of Prostate Cancer Progression." *Advances in Experimental Medicine and Biology* 399: 173–81 (1996).

Zhou, J. R., and G. L. Blackburn. "Bridging Animal and Human Studies: What Are the Missing Segments in Dietary Fat and Prostate Cancer?" *American Journal of Clinical Nutrition* 66, Suppl 6: 1572S–1580S (Dec. 1997).

CHAPTER 9:
KEEPING HIS HAIR ON HIS HEAD

Berkfeld, W. F. "Androgenetic Alopecia: An Autosomal Dominant Disorder." *The American Journal of Medicine* 98(1A): 95S–98S (Jan. 16, 1995).

Blakeslee, S. "Bald Facts About Male Self-Esteem: Losing Their Youthful Locks Triggers Profound Anxiety in Some Men." *American Health* 10(7): 24 (Sept. 1991).

Cabanac, M., and H. Brinnel. "Beards, Baldness, and Sweat Secretion." *European Journal of Applied Physiology* 58(1–2): 39–46 (1988).

Cash, T. F. "The Psychological Effects of Androgenetic Alopecia in Men." *Journal of the Academy of Dermatology* 26(6): 926–31 (June 1992).

Cipriani, R., et al. "Sex Hormone-Binding Globulin and Saliva Testosterone Levels in Men with Androgenetic Alopecia." *British Journal of Dermatology* 109(3): 249–52 (Sept. 1983).

Giralt, M., et al. "Glutathione, Glutathione S-Transferase and Reactive Oxygen Species of Human Scalp Sebaceous Glands in Male Pattern Baldness." *Journal of Investigative Dermatology* 107(2): 154–58 (Aug. 1996).

Gittleman, A. L. *Super Nutrition for Men and the Women Who Love Them.* New York: M. Evans and Company, 1996.

Goldman, B. E., D. M. Fisher, and S. L. Ringler. "Transcutaneous PO2 of the Scalp in Male Pattern Baldness: A New Piece to the Puzzle." *Plastic and Reconstructive Surgery* 97(6): 1109–16 (May 1996).

Gray, A., et al. "Age, Disease, and Changing Sex Hormone Levels in Middle-Aged Men: Results of the Massachusetts Male Aging Study." *Journal of Clinical Endocrinology and Metabolism* 73(5): 1016–25 (Nov. 1991).

Guiteras, P., M.D. "Can Bald Heads Grow Hair Again? An Update." *Executive Health Report* 27(7): 2–4 (April 1991).

Hamalainen, E., et al. "Serum Lipoproteins, Sex Hormones and Sex Hormone Binding Globulin in Middle-Aged Men of Different Physical Fitness and Risk of Coronary Heart Disease." *Atherosclerosis* 67(2–3): 155–62 (Oct. 1987).

Hochwald, L. "Better Hair from Within." *Natural Health:* 50–53 (Jan.–Feb. 1996).

Jaworski, C., A. M. Kligman, and G. F. Murphy. "Characterization of Inflammatory Infiltrates in Male Pattern Alopecia: Implications for Pathogenesis." *British Journal of Dermatology* 127(3): 239–46 (Sept. 1992).

Kaufman, K. D. "Androgen Metabolism As It Affects Hair Growth in Androgenetic Alopecia." *Dermatology Clinics* 14(4): 697–711 (Oct. 1996).

Knussmann, R., K. Christiansen, and J. Kannmacher. "Relations Between Sex Hormone Level and Characters of Hair and Skin in Healthy Young Men." *American Journal of Physical Anthropology* 88(1): 59–67 (May 1992).

Lee, K. S., K. B. Myung, and H. I. Kook. "A Clinical Study of Topical Mucopolysaccharides and Polydeoxyribonucleoprotein (Foltene) Therapy in Alopecia." *Journal of the Korean Medical Sciences* 2(3): 157–65 (Sept. 1987).

Lee, M. S., et al. "Quantification of Hair Follicle Parameters Using Computer Image Analysis: A Comparison of Androgenetic Alopecia with Normal Scalp Biopsies." *Australasian Journal of Dermatology* 36(3): 143–47 (Aug. 1995).

Miles, K. "Beautiful Hair, Skin, and Nails." *Energy Times:* 21–26 (March 1996).

Pitts, R. L. "Serum Elevation of Dehydroepiandosterone Sulfate Associated with Male Pattern Baldness in Young Men." *Journal of the American Academy of Dermatology* 16(3 pt 1): 571–73 (March 1987).

Randall, V. A. "Role of 5-Alpha-Reductase in Health and Disease." *Baillieres Clinical Endocrinology and Metabolism* 8(2): 405–31 (April 1994).

Randall, V. A., N. A. Hibberts, and K. Hamada. "A Comparison of the Culture and Growth of Dermal Papilla Cells from Hair Follicles from Non-Balding and Balding (Androgenetic Alopecia) Scalp." *British Journal of Dermatology* 134(3): 437–44 (March 1996).

Sawaya, M. E., L. S. Honig, and S. L. Hsia. "Increased Androgen Binding Capacity in Sebaceous Glands in Scalp of Male-Pattern Baldness." *Journal of Investigative Dermatology* 92(1): 91–95 (Jan. 1989).

Sawaya, M. E., and V. H. Price. "Different Levels of 5-Alpha-Reductase Type I and II, Aromatase, and Androgen Receptor in Hair Follicles of Women and Men with Androgenetic Alopecia." *Journal of Investigative Dermatology* 109(3): 296–300 (Sept. 1997).

Schmidt, J. B., A. Lindmaier, and J. Spona. "Hormonal Parameters in Androgenetic Hair Loss in the Male." *Dermatologica* 182(4): 214–17 (1991).

van der Willigen, A. H., et al. "A Preliminary Study of the Effect of 11 a-Hydroxyprogesterone on the Hair Growth in Men Suffering from Androgenetic Alopecia." *Acta Dermatologica Venereologica* 67(1): 82–85 (1987).

Young, J. W., et al. "Cutaneous Immunopathology of Androgenetic Alopecia." *Journal of the American Osteopathic Association* 91(8): 765–71 (Aug. 1991).

CHAPTER 10:
LASER SURGERY ISN'T JUST FOR WOMEN

Alster, T. S., and S. Garg. "Treatment of Facial Rhytides with a High-Energy Pulsed Carbon Dioxide Laser." *Plastic and Reconstructive Surgery* 98(5): 791–94 (Oct. 1996).

Bernstein, L. J., et al. "The Short- and Long-Term Side Effects of Carbon Dioxide Laser Resurfacing." *Dermatologic Surgery* 23(7): 519–25 (July 1997).

Nanni, C. A., and T. S. Alster. "Complications of Carbon Dioxide Laser Resurfacing. An Evaluation of 500 Patients." *Dermatologic Surgery* 24(3): 315–20 (March 1998).

Stuzin, J. M., et al. "Histologic Effects of the High-Energy Pulsed CO_2 Laser on Photoaged Facial Skin." *Plastic and Reconstructive Surgery* 99(7): 2036–50 (June 1997).

Weinstein, C., O. M. Ramirez, and J. N. Pozner. "Postoperative Care Following CO_2 Laser Resurfacing: Avoiding Pitfalls." *Plastic and Reconstructive Surgery* 100(7): 1855–66 (Dec. 1997).

CHAPTER 11:
KEEPING THE BLOOD VESSELS CLEAR AND STRONG

Adams, M. R., et al. "Oral L-Arginine Improves Endothelium-Dependent Dilatation and Reduces Monocyte Cell Adhesion to Endothelial Cells in Young Men with Coronary Artery Disease." *Atherosclerosis* 129: 261–69 (1997).

Adler, A. J., and B. J. Holub. "Effect of Garlic and Fish Oil Supplementation on Serum Lipid and Lipoprotein Concentrations in Hypercholesterolemic Men." *American Journal of Clinical Nutrition* 65: 445–50 (1997).

Austin, S. "Progress in the B Vitamin-Homocysteine-Vascular Disease Link." *Quarterly Review of Natural Medicine:* 311–12 (Winter 1997).

Azen, S. P., et al. "Effect of Supplementary Antioxidant Vitamin Intake on Carotid Arterial Wall Intima-Media Thickness in a Controlled Clinical Trial of Cholesterol Lowering." *Circulation* 94: 2369–72 (1996).

Bostom, A. G., et al. "Elevated Plasma Lipoprotein(a) and Coronary Heart Disease in Men Aged 55 Years and Younger. A Prospective Study." *Journal of the American Medical Association* 276(7): 544–48 (Aug. 21, 1996).

Braverman, E., et al. *The Healing Nutrients Within.* New Canaan, Conn.: Keats Publishing, 1997.

Brevetti, G., et al. "Effect of Propionyl-L-Carnitine on Quality of Life in Intermittent Claudication." *Journal of the American College of Cardiology* 79: 777–80 (1997).

Brown, D., and S. Austin. "Hyperlipidemia and Prevention of Coronary Heart Disease." *Quarterly Review of Natural Medicine* 61–67 (Spring 1997).

Ceremuzynski, L., T. Chamiec, and K. Herbaczynska-Cedro. "Effect of Supplemental Oral L-Arginine on Exercise Capacity in Patients with Stable Angina Pectoris." *American Journal of Cardiology* 30: 331–33 (1997).

Davies, S., et al. "Age-Related Decreases in Chromium Levels in 51,665 Hair, Sweat, and Semen Samples from 40,872 Patients—Implications for the Prevention of Cardiovascular Disease and Type II Diabetes Mellitus." *Metabolism* 46: 469–73 (1997).

Dawson, E. B., et al. "Effect of Ascorbic Acid Supplementation on Blood Levels." *Journal of the American College of Nutrition* 16: 480 (1997).

Dimmeler, S., et al. "Oxidized Low-Density Lipoprotein Induces Apoptosis of Human Endothelial Cells by Activation of CPP32-Like Proteases. A Mechanistic Clue to the 'Response to Injury' Hypothesis." *Circulation* 95(7): 1760–63 (April 1, 1997).

Efendy, J. L., et al. "The Effect of the Aged Garlic Extract, 'Kyolic,' on the Development of Experimental Atherosclerosis." *Atherosclerosis* 132: 37–42 (1997).

Everson, S. A., et al. "Interaction of Workplace Demands and Cardiovascular Reactivity in Progression of Carotid Atherosclerosis: Population Based Study." *British Medical Journal* 314(7080): 553–58 (Feb. 22, 1997).

Francesca-Rasetti, M., et al. "Extracts of Ginkgo Biloba L. Leaves and Vaccinum Myrtillus L. Fruits Prevent Photoinduced Oxidation of LDL Cholesterol." *Phytomedicines* 3: 335–38 (1996/7).

Fuhrman, B., et al. "Licorice Extract and Its Major Polyphenol Glabridin Protect LDL Against Lipid Peroxidation: In Vitro and Ex Vivo Studies in Humans and in Athroscleroric Lipoprotein E-Deficient Mice." *American Journal of Clinical Nutrition* 66: 267–75 (1997).

Galley, A. F., et al. "Regulation of Nitric Oxide Synthase Activity in Cultured Human Endothelial Cells: Effects of Antioxidants." *Free Radical Biology and Medicine* 21: 97–101 (1996).

Ghidini, O., et al. "Evaluation of the Therapeutic Efficacy of L-Carnitine in Congestive Heart Failure." *International Journal of Clinical Pharmacology, Therapy, and Toxicology* 26: 217–20 (1988).

Gittleman, A. L. *Super Nutrition for Men.* New York: M. Evans and Co., 1996.

Golan, R. *Optimal Wellness*. New York: Ballantine Books, 1995.

Gomberg-Maitland, M., and W. H. Frishman. "Thyroid Hormone and Cardiovascular Disease." *American Heart Journal* 135(2 Pt 1): 187–96 (Feb. 1998).

Grundy, S. M. "Dietary Therapy in Diabetes Mellitus—Is There a Single Best Diet?" *Diabetes Care* 14: 796–801 (1991).

Hertog, M. G., E. J. M. Feskens, and D. Kromhout. "Antioxidant Flavonoids and Coronary Heart Disease Risk." *Lancet* 349: 699 (1997).

Kamarck, T. W., et al. "Exaggerated Blood Pressure Responses During Mental Stress Are Associated with Enhanced Carotid Atherosclerosis in Middle-Aged Finnish Men: Findings from the Kuopio Ischemic Heart Disease Study." *Circulation* 96(11): 3842–48 (Dec. 2, 1997).

Kritchevsky, S. B., et al. "Dietary Antioxidants and Carotid Artery Wall Thickness. The Atherosclerosis Risk in Communities (ARIC) Study." *Circulation* 92(8): 2142–50 (Oct. 15, 1995).

Liao, J. K., et al. "Oxidized Low-Density Lipoprotein Decreases the Expression of Endothelial Nitric Oxide Synthase." *Journal of Biological Chemistry* 270(1): 319–24 (Jan. 6, 1995).

Lynch, J., et al. "Moderately Intense Physical Activities and High Levels of Cardiorespiratory Fitness Reduce the Risk of Non-Insulin-Dependent Diabetes in Middle-Aged Men." *Archives of Internal Medicine* 156(12): 1307–14 (June 24, 1996).

Meydani, S. N., et al. "Vitamin E Supplementation and In Vivo Immune Response in Healthy Elderly Subjects." *Journal of the American Medical Association* 277: 1380–86 (1997).

Morel, D. W., J. K. Hessler, and G. M. Chisolm. "Low Density Lipoprotein Cytotoxicity Induced by Free Radical Peroxidation of Lipid." *Journal of Lipid Research* 24: 1070–76 (1983).

Murray, M., and J. Pizzorno. *Encyclopedia of Natural Medicine*. Rocklin, Calif.: Prima Publishing, 1991.

Nygard, O., et al. "Coffee Consumption and Plasma and Total Homocysteine: The Hordaland Homocysteine Study." *American Journal of Clinical Nutrition* 65: 136–43 (1997).

Nygard, O., et al. "Plasma Homocysteine Levels and Mortality in Patients with Coronary Artery Disease." *New England Journal of Medicine* 337: 230–36 (1997).

Pan, X. R., et al. "Effects of Diet and Exercise in Preventing Non-Insulin Dependent Diabetes Mellitus in People with Impaired Glucose Tolerance. The Da Qing IGT and Diabetes Study." *Diabetes Care* 20: 537–44 (1997).

Ramasami, S., S. Parthasarathy, and D. G. Harrison. "Regulation of Endothelial Nitric Oxide Synthase Gene Expression by Oxidized Linoleic Acid." *Journal of Lipid Research* 39(2): 268–76 (Feb. 1998).

Rath, M. *Eradicating Heart Disease.* San Francisco, Calif.: Health Now, 1993.

Salonen, J. T., et al. "Lipoprotein Oxidation and Progression of Carotid Atherosclerosis." *Circulation* 95(4): 840–45 (Feb. 18, 1997).

Seelig, M. S. "Consequences of Magnesium Deficiency on the Enhancement of Stress Reactions; Preventive and Therapeutic Implications." *Journal of the American College of Nutrition* 13(5): 429–46 (1994).

Solzbach, U., et al. "Vitamin C Improves Endothelial Dysfunction of Epicardial Coronary Arteries in Hypertensive Patients." *Circulation* 96(5): 1513–19 (Sept. 2, 1997).

Steinberg, D. "Antioxidant Vitamins and Coronary Heart Disease." *New England Journal of Medicine* 325: 1487–89 (1992).

Tayek, J. A., S. Manglik, and E. Abemayor. "Insulin Secretion, Glucose Production, and Insulin Sensitivity in Underweight and Normal Weight Cancer Patients: A Clinical Research Center Study." *Metabolism* 46: 140–45 (1997).

Ting, H. H., et al. "Vitamin C Improves Endothelium-Dependent Vasodilation in Forearm Resistance Vessels of Humans with Hypercholesterolemia." *Circulation* 95(12): 2617–22 (June 17, 1997).

Tomoda, H., et al. "Possible Prevention of Postangioplasty Restenosis by Ascorbic Acid." *American Journal of Cardiology* 78: 1284–86 (1996).

Yam, D., A. Eliraz, and E. M. Berry. "Diet and Disease—the Israeli Paradox: Possible Dangers of a High Omega-6 Polyunsaturated Fatty Acid Diet." *Israeli Journal of Medical Science* 32: 1134–43 (1996).

Zang, A., et al. "Inhibitory Effect of Jasmine Green Tea Epicatechin Isomers on LDL Oxidation." *Journal of Nutritional Biochemistry* 8: 334–40 (1997).

Ziegler, D., et al. "Alpha-Lipoic Acid in the Therapy of Diabetic Peripheral and Cardiac Autonomic Neuropathy." *Diabetes* 46, Suppl 2: 562–66 (1997).

Ziegler, D., et al. "Effects of Treatment with the Antioxidant Alpha-Lipoic Acid on Cardiac Autonomic Neuropathy in Non-Insulin Dependent Diabetic Patients." *Diabetes Care* 20: 369–73 (1997).

CHAPTER 12:
RESISTING THE DISEASES AND DEBILITIES OF AGING

Appel, R. G., A. J. Bleyer, and J. C. McCabe. "Case Report: Analgesic Nephropathy: A Soda and a Powder." *American Journal of the Medical Sciences* 310(4): 161–66 (Oct. 1995).

Basun, H., et al. "Metals and Trace Elements in Plasma and Cerebrospinal Fluid in Normal Aging and Alzheimer's Disease." *Journal of Neural Transmission—Parkinson's Disease and Dementia Section* 3(4): 231–58 (1991).

Blaylock, R. *Excitotoxins: The Taste That Kills.* Santa Fe, N. Mex.: Health Press, 1994.

Bower, B. "Stress Hormone May Speed Up Brain Aging." *Science News* 153: 263 (April 25, 1998).

Carruthers, M. *Male Menopause: Restoring Vitality and Virility.* London: HarperCollins, 1996.

Chung, S. Y., et al. "Administration of Phosphatidylcholine Increases Brain Acetylcholine Concentration and Improves Memory in Mice with Dementia." *Journal of Nutrition* 125(6): 1484–89 (June 1995).

Cutolo, M., et al. "Androgen Replacement Therapy in Male Patients with Rheumatoid Arthritis." *Arthritis and Rheumatism* 34(1): 1–5 (Jan. 1991).

Devogelaer, J. P., S. DeCooman, and C. Nagant de Deuxchaisnes. "Low Bone Mass in Hypogonadal Males. Effect of Testosterone Substitution Therapy, a Densitometric Study." *Maturitas* 15(1): 17–23 (Aug. 1992).

Diamond, J. *Male Menopause.* Naperville, Ill.: Sourcebooks Publishing, 1997.

Eriksen, E. F., M. Kassem, and K. Brixen. "Growth Hormone and Insulin-Like Growth Factors as Anabolic Therapies for Osteoporosis." *Hormone Research* 40(1–3): 95–98 (1993).

Fagiolo, U., et al. "Immune Dysfunction in the Elderly: Effect of Thymus Hormone Administration on Several In Vivo and In Vitro Immune Function Parameters." *Aging* 2(4): 347–55 (Dec. 1990).

Flemons, W. W., and W. Tsai. "Quality of Life Consequences of Sleep-Disordered Breathing." *Journal of Allergy and Clinical Immunology* 99(2): S750–56 (Feb. 1997).

Fontenele, J. B., et al. "The Analgesic and Anti-Inflammatory Effects of Shark Cartilage Are Due to a Peptide Molecule and Are Nitric Oxide (NO) System Dependent." *Biological and Pharmaceutical Bulletin* 20(11): 1151–54 (Nov. 1997).

Fontenele, J. B., et al. "Anti-Inflammatory and Analgesic Activity of a Water-Soluble Fraction from Shark Cartilage." *Brazilian Journal of Medical and Biological Research* 29(5): 643–46 (May 1996).

Golan, R. *Optimal Wellness.* New York: Ballantine Books, 1995.

Gottlieb, M. S. "Conservative Management of Spinal Osteoarthritis with Glucosamine Sulfate and Chiropractic Treatment." *Journal of Manipulative and Physiological Therapeutics* 20(6): 400–14 (July–Aug. 1997).

Grad, B. R., and R. Rozencwaig. "The Role of Melatonin and Serotonin in Aging: Update." *Psychoneuroendocrinology* 18(4): 283–95 (1993).

Gruenwald, J. "Standardized St. John's Wort Extract Clinical Monograph." *Quarterly Review of Natural Medicine:* 289–99 (Winter 1997).

Haddon, J. W. "Immunopharmacology and Immunotoxicology." *Advances in Experimental Medicine and Biology* 288: 1–11 (1991).

Harbuz, M. S., et al. "A Protective Role for Testosterone in Adjuvant-Induced Arthritis." *British Journal of Rheumatology* 34(12): 1117–22 (Dec. 1995).

Hedman, M., E. Nilsson, and B. de la Torre. "Low Blood and Synovial Fluid Levels of Sulpho-Conjugated Steroids in Rheumatoid Arthritis." *Clinical and Experimental Rheumatology* 10(1): 25–50 (Jan.–Feb. 1992).

Hudgel, D. W. "Treatment of Obstructive Sleep Apnea: A Review." *Chest* 109(5): 1346–58 (May 1996).

Itil, T. M., et al. "Comparing the CNS Effects of *Ginkgo biloba* Extract and Tacrine in Patients with Mild to Moderate Dementia." Abstract of a presentation at the annual NCDEU Meeting of the National Institutes of Mental Health, May 28–31, 1996.

Iznucchi, S. E., and R. J. Robbins. "Clinical Review 61: Effects of Growth Hormone on Human Bone Biology." *Journal of Clinical Endocrinology and Metabolism* 79(3): 691–94 (Sept. 1994).

Jacques, P., L. Chylack. "Epidemiologic Evidence of a Role for the Antioxidant Vitamins and Carotenoids in Cataract Prevention." *American Journal of Clinical Nutrition* 53, Suppl 1: 352S–355S (Jan. 1993).

Jefferies, W. McK. *Safe Uses of Cortisone.* Springfield, Ill.: Charles C. Thomas Publishers, 1981.

Johansson, A. G., et al. "Effects of Growth Hormone and Insulin-Like Growth Factor I in Men with Idiopathic Osteoporosis." *Journal of Clinical Endocrinology and Metabolism* 81(1): 44–48 (Jan. 1996).

Khalsa, D. S., and C. Stauth. *Brain Longevity.* New York: Warner Books, 1997.

Kidd, P. M., and W. Dean. "Phosphatidylserine: The Remarkable Brain Cell Nutrient." *Nutritional News* 11(6) (June 1997).

Le Bars, P. L., et al. "Efficacy of *Ginkgo biloba* Extract for Dementia Demonstrated in One-Year Study." *JAMA* 278: 1327–32 (1997).

Lissoni, P., et al. "A Randomised Study with Subcutaneous Low-Dose Interleukin 2 Alone vs. Interleukin 2 plus the Pineal Neurohormone Melatonin in Advanced Solid Neoplasms Other Than Renal Cancer and Melanoma." *British Journal of Cancer* 69(1): 196–99 (Jan. 1994).

Lissoni, P., et al. "Role of the Pineal Gland in the Control of Macrophage Functions and Its Possible Implication in Cancer: A Study of Interactions Between Tumor Necrosis Factor-Alpha and the Pineal Hormone Melatonin." *Journal of Biological Regulators and Homeostatic Agents* 8(4): 126–29 (Oct.–Dec. 1994).

Lupien, S., et al. "Basal Cortisol Levels and Cognitive Deficits in Human Aging." *Journal of Neuroscience* 14(5 Pt 1): 2893–903 (May 1994).

Martens, H. F., et al. "Decreased Testosterone Levels in Men with Rheumatoid Arthritis: Effects of Low Dose Prednisone Therapy." *Journal of Rheumatology* 21(8): 1427–31 (Aug. 1994).

Mateo, L., et al. "Sex Hormone Status and Bone Mineral Density in Men with Rheumatoid Arthritis." *Journal of Rheumatology* 22(8): 1455–60 (Aug. 1995).

McCarthy, D. M. "Mechanisms of Mucosal Injury and Healing: The Role of Non-Steroidal Anti-Inflammatory Drugs." *Scandinavian Journal of Gastroenterology* 208, Suppl: 24–29 (1995).

McCarty, F. "The Neglect of Glucosamine as a Treatment for Osteoarthritis—A Personal Perspective." *Medical Hypotheses* 42(5): 323–27 (May 1994).

McEwen, B. S., and A. M. Magarinos. "Stress Effects on Morphology and Function of the Hippocampus." *Annals of the New York Academy of Sciences* 821: 271–84 (June 21, 1997).

Olanow, C. W., and G. W. Arendash. "Metals and Free Radicals in Neurodegeneration." *Current Opinion in Neurology* 7(6): 548–58 (Dec. 1994).

Pauling, Linus. *How to Live Longer and Feel Better.* New York: Avon Books, 1986.

Pfohl-Leszkowicz, A., et al. "High Levels of DNA Adducts in Human Colon Are Associated with Colorectal Cancer." *Cancer Research* 55(23): 5611–16 (Dec. 1, 1995).

Pipitone, V. R. "Chondroprotection with Chondroitin Sulfate." *Drugs Under Experimental and Clinical Research* 17(1): 3–7 (1991).

Pizzorno, J. *Total Wellness.* Rocklin, Calif.: Prima Publishing, 1998.

Radford, M. G., Jr., et al. "Reversible Membranous Nephropathy Associated with the Use of Non-Steroidal Inflammatory Drugs." *JAMA* 276: 466–69 (1996).

Sakai, M., H. Yamatoya, and S. Kudo. "Pharmacological Effects of Phosphatidylserine Enzymatically Synthesized from Soybean Lecithin on Brain Functions in Rodents." *Journal of Nutritional Science and Vitaminology* 42(1): 47–54 (Feb. 1996).

Seddon, J. M., et al. "Dietary Carotenoids, Vitamin A, C and E and Advanced Age-Related Macular Degeneration." *JAMA* 272: 1413–20 (1994).

Seeman, E. "Osteoporosis in Men." *Baillieres Clinical Rheumatology* 11(3): 613–29 (Aug. 1997).

Stanley, H. L., et al. "Does Hypogonadism Contribute to the Occurrence of a Minimal Trauma Hip Fracture in Elderly Men?" *Journal of the American Geriatric Society* 39(8): 766–71 (Aug. 1991).

Steward, A., and D. R. Bayley. "Effects of Androgens in Models of Rheumatoid Arthritis." *Agents and Actions* 35(3–4): 268–72 (March 1992).

Trainin, N. "Prospects of AIDS Therapy by Thymic Humoral Factor, a Thymic Hormone." *Natural Immunity and Cell Growth Regulation* 9(3): 155–59 (1990).

Visser, J. J., and K. Hoekman. "Arginine Supplementation in the Prevention and Treatment of Osteoporosis." *Medical Hypotheses* 45(3): 339–42 (Nov. 1994).

Williams, P. J., R. H. Jones, and T. W. Rademacher. "Reduction in the Incidence and Severity of Collagen-Induced Arthritis in DBA/1 Mice, Using Exogenous Dehydroepiandrosterone." *Arthritis & Rheumatism* 40(5): 907–11 (May 1997).

CHAPTER 13:
DIETARY STRATEGIES FOR STAYING POWER

Atkins, R. C., M.D. *Dr. Atkins' New Diet Revolution.* New York: M. Evans and Company, 1992.

Blankenhorn, D. H., et al. "The Influence of Diet on the Appearance of New Lesions in Human Coronary Arteries." *Journal of the American Medical Association* 263(12): 1646–52 (March 23/30, 1990).

"Entering a High-Protein Twilight Zone." *Tufts University Diet and Nutrition Letter* 14(3): 4–6 (May 1996).

Golay, A., et al. "Weight-Loss with Low or High Carbohydrate Diet?" *International Journal of Obesity and Related Metabolic Disorders* 20(12): 1067–72 (Dec. 1996).

Gudmand-Hoyer, E. "The Clinical Significance of Disaccharide Maldigestion." *American Journal of Clinical Nutrition* 59, Suppl 3: 735S–741S (March 1994).

Jacobs, R. "New Diet, Same Old Snake Oil." *Vegetarian Times* 235: 22 (March 1997).

Levy, Y., et al. "Consumption of Eggs with Meals Increases the Susceptibility of Human Plasma and Low-Density Lipoprotein to Lipid Peroxidation." *Annals of Nutrition & Metabolism* 40(5): 243–51 (1996).

Liener, I. E. "Possible Adverse Effects of Soybean Anticarcinogens." *Journal of Nutrition* 125, Suppl 3: 744S–750S (March 1995).

Marston, W. "The New Diet Food: High-Protein Diets Really Do Make You Lose Fat; That's Where the Problems Start." *Health* 10(5): 98–102 (Sept. 1996).

Masoro, E. J. "Possible Mechanisms Underlying the Antiaging Actions of Caloric Restriction." *Toxicology and Pathology* 24(6): 738–41 (Nov.–Dec. 1996).

Masoro, E. J. "Retardation of Aging Processes by Food Restriction: An Experimental Tool." *American Journal of Clinical Nutrition* 55: 1250S–1252S (1992).

McCord, H. "Meat, Milk, and Bones." *Prevention* 49(9): 51 (Sept. 1997).

Nelson, J. F., et al. "Neuroendocrine Involvement in Aging: Evidence from Studies of Reproductive Aging and Caloric Restriction." *Neurobiology of Aging* 16(5): 837–43, 855–56 (Sept.–Oct. 1995).

Norris, E. "High-Protein Diets: Where's the Beef?" *Harvard Health Letter* 22(3): 1–3 (Jan. 1997).

Oshi, F. A., and D. M. Paige. "Cow's Milk Is a Good Food for Some and a Poor Choice for Others: Eliminating the Hyperbole." *Archives of Pediatric and Adolescent Medicine* 148: 104–7 (Jan. 1994).

Plotnick, G. D., M. C. Corretti, and R. A. Vogel. "Effect of Antioxidant Vitamins on the Transient Impairment of Endothelium-Dependent Brachial Artery Vasoactivity Following a Single High-Fat Meal." *JAMA* 278(20): 1682–86 (Nov. 26, 1997).

Rao, D. R., et al. "Prevalence of Lactose Maldigestion. Influence of Age, Race, and Sex." *Digestive Diseases & Sciences* 39(7): 1519–24 (July 1994).

Schnohr, P., et al. "Egg Consumption and High-Density-Lipoprotein Cholesterol." *Journal of Internal Medicine* 235(3): 249–51 (March 1994).

Sebastian, A., et al. "Improved Mineral Balance and Skeletal Metabolism in Postmenopausal Women Treated with Potassium Bicarbonate." *The New England Journal of Medicine* 330(25): 1776–81 (June 23, 1994).

Thomas, D. "Dangerous Dieting: Weight-Loss Fads Can Be Hazardous to the Health." *Maclean's* 110(6): 54 (Feb. 10, 1997).

Vorster, H. H., et al. "Dietary Cholesterol—The Role of Eggs in the Prudent Diet." *South African Medical Journal* 85(4): 253–56 (April 1995).

Weaver, C., et al. "Calcium Bioavailability and Its Relation to Osteoporosis." *Journal of the Society for Experimental Biology and Medicine* 200: 157–60 (1992).

Weindruch, R. "The Retardation of Aging by Caloric Restriction: Studies in Rodents and Primates." *Toxicology and Pathology* 24(6): 742–45 (Nov.–Dec. 1996).

Whitten, P. L., et al. "Potential Adverse Effects of Phytoestrogens." *Journal of Nutrition* 125, Suppl 3: 771S–776S (March 1995).

Wing, R. R., J. A. Vazquez, and C. M. Ryan. "Cognitive Effects of Ketogenic Weight-Reducing Diets." *International Journal of Obesity & Related Metabolic Disorders* 19(11): 811–16 (Nov. 1995).

Yudkin, J. S. "How Can We Best Prolong Life? Benefits of Coronary Risk Factor Reduction in Non-Diabetic and Diabetic Subjects." *British Medical Journal* 306(6888): 1313–18 (May 15, 1993).

Index

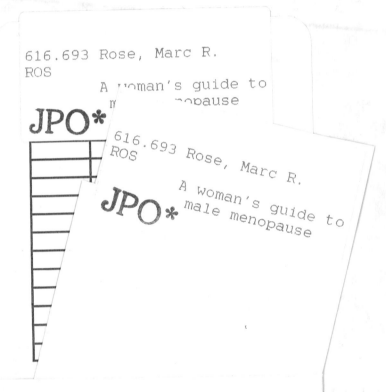

**UPPER CUMBERLAND
REGIONAL LIBRARY
208 EAST MINNEAR STREET
COOKEVILLE, TN 38501**

DEMCO